MW01485202

Obvious Parenting

Seven Simple Keys to Supporting Wellness

Ben Jessen MMS, PA-C

Cut to the Chase Communication, LLC

Obvious Parenting:
Seven Simple Keys to Supporting Wellness

Published by Cut to the Chase Communication, LLC

ISBN 978-1-7327098-0-5

Book design by LaVonne Ewing

To all the families (including my own)
who have allowed me to be a part
of their journey.

Through their struggles and their successes,
they have provided me with valuable insight
about what it truly means to be
healthy and happy.

Reviews

"I've read many general pediatric books in my nearly 40-year career as a general pediatric practitioner, and I rank this one at the top for its thorough, reader-friendly, loving, preventative approach to caring for children (and oneself) by leading a life based on strong, common sense, holistic values so often lacking in today's world. This is a perfect road-map for new and even experienced parents!"

DEAN PRINA, MD – PEDIATRICIAN

"*Obvious Parenting* reminds us of many important aspects of parenting that may be 'obvious' but are often dismissed or set aside in our hectic lives. This book teaches and reminds us of the heart of parenting and raising healthy children in today's busy world. Ben's straight-forward and to-the-point writing style allows this book to be a quick read and a go-to reference for parents and providers alike."

EMILY GRANATH, MD – PARENT & PEDIATRICIAN

"Ben Jessen's book is unlike any other parenting book. It is an easy read for busy parents, and presents information in an authentic and intuitive way by going back to the basics of healthy living. This gem offers simple truths from his own admirable journey as a father and health care provider."

ARA HAUPT, PA-C & NEW MOTHER

"Every parent-to-be needs to read this book. It is informative, but not overwhelming. It gives light to the subjects all parents need to know, from conception through adulthood, and reminds me how important it is to teach our children to take care of planet earth. *Obvious Parenting* is a book that even an experienced mom of four, like myself, can learn from!"

CHARLA B., MOTHER OF FOUR

Contents

Part Two: The Stages of Development

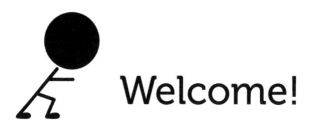

Welcome!

If you picked up this book you are probably wondering what is so obvious about parenting? With all the expectations we place on ourselves and all the information and opinions floating around, parenting seems far from obvious. In fact, more often than not, parenting, or the just the thought of parenting, can feel downright overwhelming.

Well I have good news! Parenting may not be easy, but it can be obvious. We just have to get back to the basics. Our number one job as parents is to raise healthy, happy, confident, safe and fun-loving human beings. And all we need to make this happen are seven simple keys to supporting their wellness. These keys open our thoughts and actions to prevention, and the sooner we practice prevention, the more powerful it is.

As a pediatric physician assistant and parent of two wonderful (in my humble opinion) children, I have found that the majority of pediatric books only talk about how to treat or react to a problem instead of focusing on supporting wellness and prevention. Our fast-paced culture, with its endless pressure to keep up with the Joneses, has caused significant stress on our society, health care system and the environment. By being intentional with wellness throughout all stages of life, the world will be a less stressful place for you, your family and society.

Supporting wellness requires a holistic approach toward

parenting. We must focus on our body, mind, spirit and also the environment we live in. Each of the seven universal keys discussed in this book is connected to the next. By unlocking one area of wellness, we make it easier to unlock the rest. For example, by exercising on a regular basis (second key) we are able to sleep better (fourth key), have an improved mental state (third key), and reduce the risk of injury by building strength and coordination (sixth key). Fortunately, this works for parents as well as the children they are raising.

This book starts by explaining the seven simple keys to obvious parenting. These keys are then applied to each stage of child development, from pregnancy through the teenage years. This information comes from my own personal and medical experience, the knowledge of my colleagues, and the recommendations of major medical organizations and spiritual leaders. My goal is not to be controversial, but to explain the universal basics in a fun and concise way.

A few things this book does not do. This book doesn't cover issues after they pop up; it is not a book about treatment. This book doesn't go into all the little nuances of child development. There are plenty of resources available that cover every stage of child development. Obvious parenting was written to be a quick guide to keeping your family healthy through the power of prevention.

You are on an incredible journey that will be filled with joys and challenges. These seven keys will provide a strong framework to ensure that wellness permeates your life and the life of your children.

I wish you a parenting journey filled with
health and happiness!
Ben Jessen MMS, PA-C

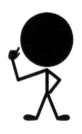

Become PROACTIVE instead of REACTIVE

We live in a reactive society. We wait for things to go bad and then deal with the aftermath. We react to over-spending with a market crash instead of living within our means and not letting greed guide our personal and business decisions. When there is a drought we limit water use during that time instead of learning to conserve water use all year round. We respond to obesity by spending billions of dollars on weight loss products instead of maintaining a healthy weight and an active life style. Being reactive may seem easier than being proactive, but making the decision to not be preemptive does have consequences! These effects can manifest themselves immediately or take years to show up.

The United States spent more than $2 trillion in 2010 on total health care, much of that on preventable diseases. Obesity alone costs America $40 billion per year! If any health care system is to work in a cost-effective manner, the population it serves needs to be healthier than ours by taking preventative measures. Not only does one decision to live an unhealthy and reactive life affect that individual, but that single choice impacts all those who participate in our health care system. We have to work together to create a system that prevents disease in the first place!

Being proactive means taking positive action every day by maintaining a healthy life balance. Taking action may seem more difficult than waiting to react but in the long run being proactive is easier. Reactive behavior is ever changing and stressful; being proactive involves practicing and eventually mastering healthy lifestyle patterns, trusting that what we do today will positively affect our future. The earlier we start our children on a path of preventive behavior the more effective our efforts will be. All it takes is a little knowledge that you put into action and repeat!

Here are two quick examples of the power of prevention.

Cancer

According to the World Health Organization (WHO) over half of cancers can be prevented through lifestyle changes. Here are a few life style choices that can drastically reduce the risk of getting cancer.

○ **Avoid tobacco:** Just by avoiding tobacco we can reduce the yearly cancer death rate by 20 percent and the overall lung cancer rate by 70 percent.

○ **Maintain a healthy weight:** Just by keeping an appropriate weight for our height (BMI) we can reduce the risk of getting cancer by approximately 20 percent.

○ **Limit alcohol use:** For all the men out there, we can reduce our risk of getting oral cancer by more than 72 percent by limiting alcohol consumption.

○ **Eat more fiber:** We can reduce all types of bowel cancer by 5 percent for each 10 grams of fiber we add to our diet.

○ **Reduce air pollution:** We can reduce the risk of cancer by up to 4 percent by reducing the exposure to air pollution.

○ **Watch your sun exposure:** We can reduce the risk for almost all skin cancers by taking appropriate sun exposure precautions.

We can decrease our family's chance of getting cancer by 50 percent just by following the seven simple keys to supporting wellness!

Heart Disease

At least 80 percent of heart disease (coronary heart disease, hypertension and stroke) is preventable according to the World Health Organization. Here are a few facts to keep in mind.

○ High blood pressure, high cholesterol and smoking are the top three risk factors.

○ Other preventable risk factors include poor diet, physical inactivity, obesity, diabetes and excessive alcohol consumption.

○ Heart disease costs the United States more than $200 billion a year.

○ More than one million Americans suffer heart attacks and strokes each year.

By becoming an obvious parent, which includes eating healthy, getting exercise, avoiding smoking, watching our weight, blood sugar and cholesterol levels, we can reduce our family's risk of having heart disease by 80 percent!

Let's pause a moment to let this powerful truth sink in.

We, as parents, have the incredible opportunity to decrease our family's cancer risk by 50 percent and heart disease risk by 80 percent. Yes, the responsibility is huge, but the rewards are SO WORTH the effort!

Part One

Seven Keys to Supporting Wellness

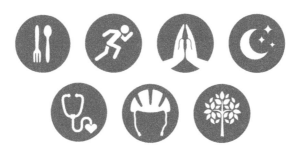

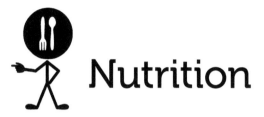 # Nutrition

It is **obvious** we want to feed our family the right stuff.

Unless you are a robot, you were born with a completely organic body designed to be fueled by nature. Unfortunately, our fast-paced society has altered our nutritional course from one of natural fuels to processed foods in order to make it more convenient for "families on the go." Thankfully, we are starting to focus on nature once again. Some food packages are now labeled with "made with all natural ingredients." Should we be alarmed that manufacturers find it necessary to label their foods "all natural?" If it is not natural, then what is it? When we take a look at the ingredients list we quickly find out.

Label Reading

Almost every food we buy will have an **Ingredients List** and a **Nutrition Facts Label**. These labels are required by the Food and Drug Administration (FDA) to help us know what we are putting in our bodies.

Ingredients List

The FDA requires an ingredients label on all packages, listing the ingredients from greatest quantity to least quantity. For example, if sugar is the first ingredient on the list, you want to limit your intake of that food. Additionally, if you read ingredients you have never heard of, ideally you would find out what they are before allowing your family to eat them. A great place to start reading labels is at home with food you have already bought. For the past decade I have researched many ingredients I did not recognize. Some of the ingredients I looked up were found to be safe but the effects of others were downright scary! When your family is involved, you will discover that it is much easier to purchase foods with shorter lists of mostly natural ingredients.

Which foods have the shortest ingredient labels? Everything in the produce section. The only ingredient in an apple is "apple." Of course there are plenty of products that have only one or a few ingredients that are not good for you—like sugar. But obvious parenting tells us that an apple is a better option than a bag of sugar.

Looking at every ingredient is a great habit to develop. Take time to read ingredients labels and you will feel confident when you are at the checkout stand, knowing the health value of every item in your cart. A few quick rules on ingredients label reading:

○ The shorter the list, the better. For example, it is possible to buy peanut butter that has one ingredient: peanuts. You don't need the added fat, sugar and salt found in most peanut butter.

○ Make it easy! Try buying foods that don't require an ingredients label at all, like fruits and vegetables.

○ Especially read labels on food you haven't purchased before.

○ The ingredients are listed from the greatest amount to least, so if sugar is one of the first three ingredients, limit that food.

○ Avoid foods with partially hydrogenated, hydrogenated, or trans-fats in them. Do not be fooled by the "no trans-fat per serving" label on the front of the package because it still may contain processed fats.

TO LEARN MORE ABOUT TRANS FATS:

www.fda.gov/food/ucm292278.htm

Nutrition Facts Label

The Nutrition Facts label tells you the serving size, calories, and nutrients in each serving. Many diet plans are based on the Nutrition Facts label and recommend consuming only this much fat and protein, or that many carbohydrates and calories. I believe these types of plans take too much effort and math skill. Do not get caught up in reading the Nutrition Facts label unless recommended by your personal dietician, nutritionist, or fitness coach. What really matters is the source of those nutrients. For example, two different foods may have the same amount of carbohydrates but one comes from whole grain wheat and the other from corn syrup. Which one would be better to fuel your child with? If you are reading a Nutrition Facts label, focus on foods high in fiber and low in sugars.

TO LEARN MORE ABOUT LABEL READING:

www.fda.gov

www.healthline.com

Fruits and Vegetables

Why are we constantly encouraged to eat more fruits and vegetables? It is now recommended that we eat a total of 6 to 11 servings of fruits and vegetables per day! (A serving size is approximately the size of your fist.) The recommended number of daily servings continues to increase because studies show that fruits and vegetables are the pillars of good health and prevention. Here are a few reasons why fruits and vegetable are so great.

Phytonutrients

Fruits and vegetables contain thousands and thousands of healthy compounds called phytonutrients or phytochemicals. These wonderful compounds work synergistically with each other to form antioxidants and nutrients to help support our health and well-being. We have not been able to replicate nature's recipe for these compounds. There is no multivitamin that comes close to providing the nutrients found in fruits and vegetables. Growing evidence shows that phytonutrients have powerful preventative effects on us.

Fiber

Most Americans consume only a fraction of the daily recommended fiber. The average American consumes only 15 grams of fiber per day when the recommendation is 25 to 38 grams. Fiber's main purpose is to keep our bowels moving and our stools (not the ones we sit on) soft. Soluble fiber is a type of fiber that helps keep our bowel movements soft by trapping water in its structure. Insoluble fiber helps move the stool along by not dissolving. Allowing waste to get backed up causes constipation and increases the risk of colon cancer, diverticulitis, irritable bowel syndrome, and chronic abdominal pain. Certain fibers also help maintain a balanced probiotic population in our gut. Fiber's other important role is to slow the absorption of sugar. When sugar is absorbed too fast it stresses our pancreas. It also gives our kids a sugar rush that we all enjoy, especially on long car rides or right before bed (just kidding!). Fruits and vegetables are a great source of fiber. Other good sources are whole grains and legumes (beans, lentils, peas and peanuts).

Complex Carbohydrates

Fruits and vegetables break down into complex carbohydrates. These are the "good carbs"...slowly digested forms of energy that also contain vitamins, minerals and fiber. These should replace the "bad carbs" like table sugar, candy, honey, fruit juice and soft drinks. These simple carbohydrates can stress our systems and increase caloric consumption too quickly. This can lead to tooth decay, obesity and all the bad things that go with it.

Protein

Proteins are the building blocks for our cells and thus all the tissues in our body. Proteins are made from amino acids. Most amino acids are produced by our bodies and are considered non-essential, meaning they are not essential to find in our diet. Some amino acids cannot be made by our bodies so we must get them from the foods we eat. These are called essential amino acids. Vegetables, whole grains, beans, nuts, and meats are excellent sources of essential amino acids. Believe it or not, a vegetarian based diet can include all the essential amino acids we need to build a strong and healthy body. Meat is optional for a diet rich in protein.

Food Enzymes

Raw fruits and vegetables contain their own enzymes that are activated when we eat them. These enzymes help break down food, making them more easily digestible. The natural enzymes found in plants help decrease the need for our bodies to produce their own digestive enzymes. This puts less stress on our digestive systems and allows more nutrients to be absorbed. Beginning a meal with a salad has been common practice for centuries because we instinctively know it helps us prime our digestive system for the rest of the meal. Over-heating food can destroy these enzymes. We heat food to make it softer and easier to chew but in doing so we sacrifice the natural power of enzymes. Of course it is enjoyable to eat a hot meal, but we should try to have raw fruits and vegetables with every meal as well.

Fats

We are often told to limit our fat intake because fat is one of the most calorie-dense nutrients. However, there are good fats and bad fats so it is important to know the difference. Plants provide some of the best fats for our bodies. Healthy fats include monounsaturated and polyunsaturated fats. These types of fat actually help reduce cholesterol, inflammation and heart disease. Good sources of healthy fats include avocados, nuts, seeds, most plant based oils, eggs, and fish. On the other hand, saturated fats from animal products and trans-fats (hydrogenated oils) can be harmful to our bodies. There is enough evidence to recommend avoiding all trans-fats (hydrogenated oils) and to limit or avoid saturated fats, especially from red meat. Decreasing saturated fats has been shown to decrease LDL (bad cholesterol) levels, thus decreasing the risk of heart disease and inflammation.

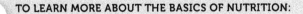

TO LEARN MORE ABOUT THE BASICS OF NUTRITION:

www.choosemyplate.gov

https://my.clevelandclinic.org/
articles/11208-fat-what-you-need-to-know

Grains

Just like fruits and vegetables, enjoying a variety of grains is a healthy way to eat. Some examples include wheat, rice, corn, millet, amaranth, quinoa, arrowroot and buckwheat. Each type of grain contains different beneficial nutrients. Avoid products made with refined grains (white flower, white rice) that have been stripped of their bran and germ. The bran and germ portions of the grain contain all the good stuff including magnesium, selenium, copper and manganese. Look for products that include whole grains on their ingredients label.

Gluten

Gluten is a natural binding agent found in wheat, barley, rye, and triticale. If you have ever made paper mache or play-dough out of white flour, you have seen gluten in action. Many people feel that gluten can contribute to *leaky gut* (allowing larger molecules into the blood stream from the intestines, which creates an abnormal immune response). Others say they are sensitive to gluten and avoid it because it causes bloating and gas, which may actually be due to grain fermenting in the digestive system. There is a difference between being "gluten sensitive" and being diagnosed with celiac disease*. It is important to listen to your body and avoid foods that make you feel "off." Keep in mind that many foods containing gluten can be particularly nutritious. Gluten-free foods can also be nutritious, but many are highly processed, cost more, and are higher in calories. If you buy a gluten-free product make sure it is whole grain.

*When people have **celiac disease** their bodies produce an abnormal immune response when they consume gluten. This response can damage the lining of their small intestines, making it harder to absorb other nutrients. This is an under-diagnosed disease that, if ignored, can lead to severe complications. Celiac disease has a strong genetic component. Talk to your health care provider if you have a close relative diagnosed with celiac disease to see if you need to be tested.

Organic vs. Non-Organic

It would be ideal if all produce were organic* but unfortunately they are not. Pesticides* have been used for decades to prevent crops from being destroyed. The use of pesticides can help improve the yield and quality of the produce but at a potential cost to the health of the consumer and environment. Pesticides are designed to kill unwanted living pests and so they come with an inherent risk of harming other living species. Washing your produce is a good step toward protecting your family but it may not remove all pesticides. Better yet, make an effort to support organic farming by buying organic produce when available. The higher cost of organics should go down as demand increases. Growing your own produce can also help reduce your exposure to pesticides and gardening is a wonderful family activity.

***organic produce:** Grown without the use of pesticides, synthetic fertilizers, bioengineering including the use of genetically modified products, ionizing radiation and sewage sludge.

***pesticides:** Chemicals used to kill "harmful" animals and plants. May include herbicides, insecticides, fungicides, and poisons used to kill rodents.

TO LEARN MORE ABOUT
PESTICIDE LEVELS IN PRODUCE:
www.ewg.org

Animal Products

Land Meat

There are many who say our bodies were designed to eat animals. It is obvious that our bodies can handle and utilize animal products and have for thousands of years. Land animal meat is high in protein, iron, B-vitamins (especially B12), zinc, copper, and manganese along with other nutrients. However, even though animal products are high in some essential nutrients, they are not a vital part of a human diet and have potentially negative effects on our bodies when over-consumed. Ingesting too many animal products, especially red meat, is affecting our health by increasing cancer rates and heart disease. Some argue that diets high in meat and low in grains can help us lose weight and thus reduce the negative consequences of being overweight. It is true; anytime we decrease our caloric intake we will lose weight. But substituting one over-consumed food for another may not be the healthiest choice!

Many people equate animal meat with protein. I regularly see parents who worry their child is protein deficient because they can't get their toddler to eat meat. Vegetables, beans, nuts and grains are also good sources of protein. For example, per 100 calories, broccoli has more protein than beef! Four ounces of black beans have just as much protein as four ounces of ground beef. The amount of protein we need depends on our age and activity level so talk to your health care provider about how much your child needs.

If you and/or your family are vegan (consume only plants and no animal products) then make sure you are all getting enough B12 and iron, as well as protein, from other sources such as seitan (wheat gluten), tofu, tempeh, edamame, lentils, beans, nuts and seeds and fortified cereals.

Processed Meats

Growing up, my friends and I would refer to hot dogs as "lips and ass" because we heard the cheap ones we ate were made from meat scraps. It turns out we may have been right! Not only are processed meats made from multiple animal parts, but they have been shown to increase the risk of cancer. If you are going to feed your kids hot dogs or other processed meats, make sure you know what is in them and buy the most natural version of the product.

Water Meat

Here fishy-fishy! Consuming fish and other sea creatures with high amounts of omega-3 fatty acids, trace minerals and protein can be a healthy part of our diets. But we have to be responsible by purchasing seafood from companies that do not support overfishing. It is important to be aware of the way our water-dwelling friends have been harvested. Currently, more responsible fish options include Pacific cod, New Zealand salmon, tilapia, albacore tuna, trout, and Alaska crab.

Some species of fish and shellfish contain high amounts of contaminants including mercury. Fish to avoid include those big predators like shark, swordfish, and marlin because they are higher on the food chain and thus contain higher amounts of mercury. Other fish that have higher amounts of mercury include orange roughy, Chilean sea bass, grouper, monkfish and tuna so these should be limited. Cleaner fish options include salmon, pollock, butterfish, anchovies, crab and clams.

TO LEARN MORE ABOUT WHICH FISH TO EAT AND WHICH FISH ARE ENDANGERED:

www.nrdc.org

www.safinacenter.org

Dairy

It is still ingrained in many people's minds (including health care providers) that dairy is an essential part of our diet. Yes, dairy is high in calcium, potassium, calories, and trace amounts of vitamin D (milk is fortified with vitamin D.) However, these nutrients are not unique to dairy products. They are also plentiful in nuts, beans, and whole grains.

There is little evidence that the high calcium content in dairy decreases the risk of osteoporosis or fractures. A few studies have shown that a diet high in dairy products could increase the risk of prostate and ovarian cancers.

Studies have also shown that consuming dairy products may increase the risk of insulin-dependent diabetes. Lactose (the sugar in dairy products) can also cause some uncomfortable abdominal symptoms in those lacking the enzyme that breaks down that sugar.

While I do enjoy dairy products including cheese, frozen yogurt, and ice cream, I try to limit them and avoid drinking cow milk altogether. I limit my family's dairy products as well, not only for our health, but also to help the environment. Dairy farms are one of the biggest polluters in the animal agriculture industry.

We don't all have to be vegetarian or vegan, but we should be conscious about where our food comes from. Try to eat free range, grass-fed, and organic animal products that are raised more humanely. If we all reduced the amount of animal products raised for mass consumption, our bodies and the earth would be a healthier place.

TO LEARN MORE ABOUT DAIRY:

www.pcrm.org

Portion Control

It is important to pay attention to not just the food we eat but the amount we eat. For healthy portion control, we can learn to listen to our bodies so we know when we are full. Evidence shows that those who eat at the lower end of their caloric range live longer, healthier lives. This does not mean we need to deprive our bodies of the calories (energy) and nutrients we need, but be aware that excess calories can take years off our lives.

Teach your children portion control by setting a good example and not overeating. When you go out to eat, remember you can always save some for later. Before digging in, look at the amount of food on the plate and then picture it all fitting into your stomach. If you wonder how all that food is going to fit, it is probably too much. Sometimes what we feel as a hunger cue is actually our body's signal that it needs more water. The next time you or your kids are hungry after eating a large meal, put down your fork, drink some water (not soda) and wait a few minutes before consuming more food.

Hydration

Our bodies are made up of approximately 70 percent water. We are not made up of 70 percent milk, juice, sport drinks or soda. These products are made mostly from water but contain excess calories we may not need.

If possible, the majority of our fluid intake should be clean filtered water. A general rule of thumb is that we should drink enough water to have clear-looking urine every few hours.

More specific recommendations for fluid intake (based on average amounts):

○ Children 1–3 years old: 24 oz per day

○ Children 4–8 years old: 32 oz per day

○ Children 9–13 years old: 48 oz per day

○ Children 14 years old and up: 64 oz per day

Tap Water

Tap water can come from your city or from a well. Both sources of water can have contaminants in them. If you have well water, you should have it tested at least yearly. Tap water from a city or town can contain a small amount of contaminants that are potentially harmful. It is slightly disgusting to think about the recycled water we consume, considering all the chemicals and other junk we flush down our pipes. Luckily, tap water is regulated by the EPA (Environmental Protection Agency) and is regularly tested by your town.

You can find out about the safety of your water by requesting the *consumer confidence report* from your water district. EPA regulations are not perfect so please support your local clean water act.

TO LEARN MORE ABOUT THE CLEAN WATER ACT:

www.cleanwateraction.org

Water Filters

There are several types of home water filters, from above-the-sink carbon filters to whole-house reverse osmosis filters. If you are interested in filtering your water, first find out which contaminants are in it. This can be done by private water quality testing or reading the water quality report from your town. Once you know what you are up against you can find a filter that helps reduce those contaminants. At a minimum, I advise getting a carbon filter for your drinking water and replacing it as recommended by the manufacturer. However, most carbon filters are not good at removing lead, heavy metals, fluoride and microbes. This is a concern only if your water contains these contaminants.

Bottled Water

Bottled water is not as tightly regulated as tap water so some bottled water may have more contaminates than the water from your faucets. If you drink a specific brand of bottled water do some investigating and find out what is in it. Bottled water is much more expensive than tap water and adds a significant amount of waste to our environment. A much better alternative is using a glass, metal, or BPA-free water bottle and filling it up with filtered water from your home.

Fluoridation

I have had many families express concerns about fluoride in their water. Fluoride occurs naturally in our water but some communities add more when the natural fluoride content is low. Fluoride helps fight cavities by protecting and rebuilding the enamel in our teeth. Unfortunately, too much fluoride can be toxic to humans. Luckily, the amount put in our municipal water is so minimal that it should not cause any significant health concerns. If you have well water, have it tested for fluoride. The amount of fluoride in well water may be more than municipal water.

Topical fluoride is one of the best ways to get fluoride to the teeth, so using fluoride toothpaste or fluoride rinses are important as well. If you want non-fluoridated water then you will have to get a filter that is designed to take out fluoride (most of them don't) or find out if your bottled water contains it.

LEARN MORE ABOUT FLUORIDATION:
https://ilikemyteeth.org/fluoridation

Dental Care

There are multiple studies showing a link between dental health and overall health and well-being. Gum disease, especially chronic inflammation (gingivitis), may be associated with cardiac disease, memory loss, pre-term labor, and blood sugar control. Bacteria overgrowth and imbalance from not taking care of our teeth and gums actually affects our whole body!

The American Academy of Pediatric Dentists recommends that we start teeth brushing and dental visits as soon as our child's first tooth peeks through. Start using fluorinated tooth-paste once or twice a day from the beginning. Only use a smear on your child's teeth until they are three years old, then increase to a pea-size amount.

We should start flossing when there are enough teeth to floss between. We should also change our toothbrush every three to four months or sooner if the bristles look worn.

LEARN MORE ABOUT DENTAL CARE:

www.aapd.org

Supplements

Supplements are just that. They are intended to supple-ment our diet, not to replace it. Supplements are advertised as a necessary addition to everyone's life. This is not true! There is no proof that multivitamins prevent chronic diseases in most individuals. In fact, some of the longest-living and healthiest humans never take multivitamins. However, certain supple-ments can be beneficial. They may also be necessary for some people due to chronic illness or lifestyle choices.

Does it hurt to take a multivitamin every day? Most likely it won't. Most multivitamins have a small amount of several vitamins and minerals, and these small amounts are typically not toxic. But be careful, because some vitamins and minerals can become toxic if consumed in high amounts. Fat-soluble vi-tamins like vitamin A, D, E, and K, can become more concen-trated in our bodies over time because they are not excreted as quickly as water-soluble vitamins like vitamin C, and the B vitamins.

Vitamin D

Vitamin D is one supplement that makes sense for some of us to take. Studies have shown that up to 40 percent of people in the United States are deficient in vitamin D. People at greater risk of vitamin D deficiency are those with darker pigmented skin, people who are overweight, people with gastrointestinal disorders, and those who don't get enough sun.

Our bodies produce vitamin D when exposed to ultraviolet B rays from the sun. However, our society spends most of its time indoors, and when we are outside we protect ourselves from the sun with sunscreen and clothing to reduce the risk of skin cancer. If possible, we should spend about 10 minutes every day outside in the mid-day sun with our legs and arms exposed. This could give us up to 10,000 IU (international units) of vitamin D naturally.

Vitamin D is important to our health in many ways. Vitamin D helps our bodies absorb calcium and phosphorus, which reduces the risk of rickets. Vitamin D helps regulate our nervous system and helps support our immune system. It may even help to prevent heart disease and some cancers including breast, colon, and prostate. It is possible to get vitamin D from our diet but in lesser amounts. The best natural sources include fatty fish like tuna, salmon and mackerel. Vitamin D is also found in egg yolks, cheese and some mushrooms. Most of the vitamin D we receive from processed foods has been added by food manufacturers.

Probiotics

People in industrialized countries tend to live in a more sterile environment than those in second- and third-world countries. Our food is rinsed several times before we eat it. We live in cleaner homes and we consume more antibiotics from food and medication than ever before. To prevent disease, we clean and sterilize as much as possible. While there are a plethora of bugs in the environment we don't want to infect us, there are also countless bugs that are helpful to have living in our guts. Probiotics are live bacteria and yeasts that benefit our digestive system. These healthy microorganisms have been shown to help aid in digestion and the processing and production of nutrients. Probiotics may decrease leaky gut, and recent evidence shows they play a huge part in supporting our immune system. They may also play a role in preventing obesity.

It is important to keep these beneficial bugs in balance. They can become out of balance with exposure to antibiotics found in food and medications. Stress and some types of infections can also cause an imbalance. To help keep probiotics in balance we can take a probiotic supplement that contains different strains of bacteria. Those that have been studied and found to be helpful include Lactobacillus, Bifidobacteria, and a yeast probioitic Saccharomyces boulardii. Probiotic supplements are proven to help reduce diarrhea from antibiotic use and infections but other health benefits need more research. Foods containing probiotics include brined pickles, kombucha, unpasteurized sauerkraut, sourdough bread, miso, tempeh and dairy products like yogurt and kefir.

Prebioitics

Prebiotics are non-digestible carbohydrates or fiber that help the good bacteria and yeasts thrive and stay balanced in our digestive system. One of the most well-known prebiotics is inulin. Good sources of prebiotics are asparagus, artichokes, oatmeal, whole wheat, legumes, bananas and plants from the onion family.

Whole Food Supplements

Many people feel that if we don't eat enough fruits and vegetables we should take a supplement of some kind. Why not, then, take a whole food supplement that is closer nutritionally to what you feel you are lacking (whole foods) instead of a multivitamin made of synthetically derived vitamins and minerals? Theoretically, whole food supplements make sense but obvious parenting tells us they aren't as good as the real thing. Most whole food supplements deviate from the raw whole food by adding synthetic micronutrients to reach levels labeled on the products. It is difficult to compare the activity level and absorption rate of the nutrients in a supplement compared to raw unprocessed whole food. However, if you simply can't get your family to eat the real thing and want to fill in the gaps, a whole food supplement may be a good choice for you. There are several whole food supplement products on the market so be sure to choose one that is third party tested for purity and research proves its benefit.

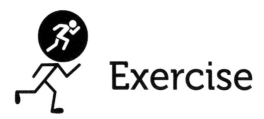

Exercise

It is **obvious** that our bodies were designed to move!

Many people hit a roadblock when they think about exercising because to them, exercise is a form of work and is not pleasurable. Exercise can easily be at the bottom of our priority list due to other pressures like work, family, TV, and housework. However, a good workout increases our energy, and thus our productivity. Exercise also improves our hormone levels and immune system function. In fact, regular exercise can decrease the risk of getting almost every chronic disease, which could save us a considerable amount of money in health care costs.

In this age of devices with big screens, small screens and all sizes in-between, we sit in our office chairs, couches, or recliners for hours, not noticing the proverbial rust building in our joints because our minds are occupied by electronics. Yet our bodies are made to be in motion, to be "one" with movement. So let's get out and move our bodies! We'll call it "movement" instead of the more daunting word, "exercise."

It doesn't matter what we do to get ourselves moving. Sometimes we have to think outside the "box" or gym to find an activity we enjoy. It doesn't have to be the same movement each day, but we should be moving daily: walk the dog instead of letting it out in the backyard. Scrub the tub. Wash the car by hand. Walk to the mail box. We should move our bodies until our hearts pound and our lungs have to work harder. Showing our children how to get physically active is one of the most important gifts we can give them. Keep in mind a common adage with a twist: A family that plays together stays *healthy* together.

Everyone has a slightly different body type. We may be good at some activities and not so good at others. This does not mean we can't use this wonderful vessel we have all been given. Humans continue to redefine what our bodies are capable of doing. Just look at how sports have evolved in the past few decades. It seems all we need is an imagination and determination to accomplish amazing physical acts. This includes those who were born with, or acquired, a change in their physical makeup. We have seen amazing achievements in the Special Olympics and Paralympics.

There is a direct connection between our bodies and our minds. When we move our muscles, we move those gears in our mind. When we feel good about the look and feel of our outer vessel, we feel good about the gift inside! Just remember that no matter how hard we move, we may never have that digitally enhanced supermodel body on the cover of a magazine. But we are no doubt healthier, more beautiful, and just as fit!

Children are pre-programmed to move. Observe how much infants move once they find out that they can get from point A to point B on their own. Look at the constant movement of toddlers whose parents can barely keep up! Even school-age children have difficulty staying still. There is growing evidence that classrooms that integrate physical activity, or more freedom to move around, perform better academically. Recess could be the most important subject of the school day!

We should try to get our kids to exercise 60 minutes per day. Three days each week their movement should be moderate to vigorous, meaning exercising hard enough to increase their heart rate and respiratory rate. Limiting the time your child spends in front of a screen will help them achieve these movement goals.

Cardiorespiratory Fitness

One of the most important muscles to train is our heart. The heart is the "king" of muscles, the controller of our destiny. We really can't train our heart without training our respiratory system, and vice versa. We call this "cardiorespiratory fitness (cardio=heart; respiratory=breath)." When we work our cardiorespiratory system through activities that increase our heart and breath rate, we make these systems more efficient at rest as well as during exercise. Multiple studies have shown that cardiorespiratory fitness increases our life span, decreases risk of diabetes, decreases cholesterol levels, lowers blood pressure, and reduces the risk of some cancers. Movement also helps strengthen our bones and may delay the progression of Alzheimer's disease. It is recommended that we work our hearts 30 minutes at a time, five days per week at a moderate intensity. Physical signs can also be clues to the intensity of our workout. For example, being able to talk but not being able to belt out our favorite song is a sign of moderate intensity. We should also be sweating after 10 minutes or so. If we want to cut that workout time in half, we will have to step up to a vigorous intensity. We know we are at a vigorous intensity by our quicker, deeper breathing, to the point where we can only say a few words at a time and are sweating after only a few minutes.

Heart Rate Goals

In people age 10 or older, the normal number of heartbeats in one minute is 60 to 100. Our maximum heart rate is calculated by subtracting our age from 220. (Example: 220 minus 40 yrs old = 180 beats per minute). Our target heart rate when we are exercising is 50–85 percent of our maximum heart rate. (Example: 180 beats per minute x 50 percent = 90 beats per minute and 180 beats per minute x 85 percent = 153 beats per minute). So a 40-year-old's target heart rate is between 90–153 beats per minute. Heart rate goals are unrealistic for kids under 10 years old, but they can be a good tool for increasing cardio-respiratory fitness in older kids and adults.

LEARN MORE ABOUT HEART RATE ZONES:
www.medicalnewstoday.com/
articles/235710.php

Strength Training

If we move our muscles enough, they will grow and get stronger. If we want our bodies to function better, we need to move and stress our muscles to help improve their efficiency. The stronger we are, the easier it is to do everyday activities. Strength training also increases bone strength, improves sleep, improves balance, decreases injury (unless you over-train), helps regulate blood sugar, and helps burn calories. The more muscle we have, the higher our metabolism is and the less likely we are to store harmful metabolites that could lead to cancer.

Being strong doesn't mean we have to be big and buff like The Rock, but it can if we want it to be! Everyone is built differently. For some people it is easy and desirable to build big, defined muscles, and for others it is not. Everyone can improve their physique at any age, but it is easier the younger we are. It is also easy to lose our muscle mass and physique at any age through laziness, stress and over-eating.

As our bodies are developing, the safest and most effective strength training is through the use of our own body weight. Our children will automatically become stronger by using their muscles as they walk, run, climb and play. To encourage further muscle development we must allow our children to try out different sports and activities. There is no reason kids should be working out on machines or using weights at the gym until they are 11 years old or older.

We should be active with our children and show them we care about how our own bodies look and move. Show them that working our bodies makes us feel better physically and mentally. Learn activities they want to learn, and play physically with them every day.

Stretching

Children are naturally more flexible than adults. We continue to be flexible through *dynamic* stretching or stretching while moving. As we grow and put more demands on our bodies, our muscles get tighter and need to be stretched more. When we get older we have a tendency to limit our range of movement. Therefore, it is important to add *static* stretching, or stretching while holding a position, to our exercise routine.

Increased flexibility improves range of motion of our joints, increases blood flow to our muscles, and decreases risk of injuries. Stretching is more productive after we warm our muscles up with light exercise. It is recommended we stretch two to three days per week depending on our sport or activity. Doing yoga as a family or just stretching in front of the TV with our children a few times a week is a worthwhile practice. A great stretch is hanging from a bar to help stretch the upper torso and back. Hamstring stretches are also important because those muscles tend to naturally tighten up and are directly linked to our backs.

LEARN MORE ABOUT STRETCHING:

www.mayoclinic.org

www.bodybuilding.com

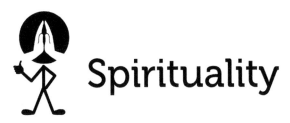 # Spirituality

> It is **obvious** we do not want to break our child's spirit!

Spirituality is a means to show us we are not alone. There is a universal connectedness that is hard to deny. There are multiple ways of expressing this concept. We use terms like God, Love, Energy, Prayer, Spirit and Karma to show our belief in that "Force" in everyone's life. We all come from the purest, most perfect power in the universe! There comes a time in most of our lives, that this belief can help get us through some rough and lonely times.

Spirituality has the power of prevention. Our spirit is directly tied to our thoughts and emotions and can control how our bodies function. The most obvious example of this is the placebo effect: when we expect a pill will help us feel better, up to 30 percent of the time it will, even if it is just a sugar pill. Another example is a spontaneous cure or remission from cancer that cannot be explained by science.

Not only can our positive thoughts improve our health, but also the health of others through the power of prayer. There are multiple studies showing the benefits of prayer in healing. We all have unlimited potential!

If you don't consider yourself as "spiritual," think of yourself as "connected." We cannot avoid being connected to other people, animals and the environment because on an atomic level, we are all made of the same atoms and we are transferring those atoms between each other all the time. As connected as we are, everyone sees the world from their own point of view.

Each individual has a special gift or ability we need to find and share for the benefit of the whole. We are all here to work as a team and to learn from one another with the common goal of making this world a beautiful place to live! Being spiritual also means practicing self-respect and respect for others, gratitude, optimism, love, and commitment.

Self-Respect/Love

Teach your children to love themselves and who they are. Having a strong sense of self-respect and love keeps our path straight. If young people are confident and self-respecting, their peers will not be able to pressure them into doing something that could harm themselves or others. Confidence and self-love reduces bullying by eliminating any sense of weakness. Believing in ourselves means we are in control of our thoughts and feelings, and others cannot control our happiness. Teach self-love through action. By showing our children we can forgive ourselves and respect our own bodies and emotions, we give them a shield of protection from those who want to put them down. Let's give our children confidence not to judge. A person with confidence is not cocky as long as they are not judging others.

Respect is a two-way street! What goes around comes around. We must teach our kids to respect others' beliefs and how to respect our Mother Earth. Kids who don't show respect for others, themselves, or the planet will not be respected by their peers. And we, as parents, are responsible for teaching this through our own everyday actions.

Oneness

It is obvious we are not alone, even if we feel that way. There are over seven billion people in this world! Each one of us is made of the same atoms and molecules that are the building blocks of every living and non-living form in the universe. This truth proves we have a connection, or oneness, with everything and everyone. This concept can be the key to unlocking our ability to forgive, to communicate, to share a bond, no matter what the circumstances. This bond can be very helpful for our children as they develop their individuality and their egos strengthen. To help them avoid loneliness, misunderstanding and frustration, we must help our children realize we are all taking this journey together! This can help them get through some difficult times.

We are never alone because the "Force" is always with us! That same energy that we all come from is powerful. Even when we are physically and mentally alone, we are always connected to the energy that drives us all. We can tap into this infinite energy by calming our mind and listening to our gut. This may sound cheesy, but it is true. When your teenagers are feeling overwhelmed by their ego and social pressures, teaching them to trust in this "Force" can save their lives and the lives of others.

Gratitude

Being grateful about life and what we have sends a message to the universe that we want more of the same. Gratitude opens us up to receiving more good! Having an attitude of gratitude for every bad or good experience helps us to keep a positive and powerful outlook. It can prevent us from falling into the "poor me" point of view. Even if we are having a rough day, there is always something to be grateful for. It can be as simple as the food we eat for breakfast, or the bed we sleep in. Growing up, we have a lot of days that push us beyond our comfort zone and leave us with a mind full of frustration and confusion. Evening is a good time to practice clearing our minds of these frustrations so we may go to sleep with final thoughts of gratitude. We will wake up with a refreshed mind because thankful energy and thoughts are healing. Gratitude also cancels out worry! By filling our minds with what we are thankful for, not what we are worrying about, we will help prevent anxiety and depression.

Optimism

Optimism and gratitude are best friends. When we are grateful, we tend to have an optimistic view on life. We can teach our kids to wake up with optimism by waking up happy ourselves! Be grateful for what we already enjoy and what we are about to enjoy! If we show our children how to be excited for the day to come they will see that every day is a gift! Yes, we will face pain, frustration, and challenges. But we can use optimism as a positive force to get through them. If a kid says, "Life sucks!" they need an optimism intervention. It is one thing to say it, but another to believe it. Help them to draw on their internal reserve of optimism to overcome their negative feelings.

Love

Love is the universal glue that positively binds everything together. Love can be thought of as the spirit or force that powers positive action. The pure, unconditional love children have is a feeling that every parent never forgets! I'll never forget the way my boys showed me unconditional love when they were toddlers. Out of nowhere, they would hold my face gently in their tiny little hands and gaze into my eyes with the purest look of peace, joy, and love. Then they'd plant a big sloppy kiss somewhere on my face. This pure love is something we should give back to our children. There are many ways to show love, but the most simple and powerful way to show our love is by giving our time. Do not be afraid to feel and give LOVE!

Time

Our love/hate relationship with time will never end! Unaware of the future, children make time stand still by focusing only on the present moment. They truly know how to live in the here and now. Then they become older and suffer through times of boredom when they wish the clock ticked faster. During adulthood there are days when we wish time would slow down so we can get everything done. As parents, we have to balance being in the present moment and planning for the future. We cannot save time; we can only spend it. First and foremost, make time for family. Be an example as you live today, play today, learn today, and make a difference today!

Children who grow up without spending time with a mother or father have an increased risk of making unhealthy decisions, from finding friends in the wrong places and for the wrong reasons, to escaping reality with drugs and alcohol. These kids will rebel because, deep down, they feel they are not worthy of anybody's time. Be worth your children's time!

Even though we may not be focused on our children, they are often focused on us. If they respect us they will follow our lead, even when we think they are not watching. We are all human and make mistakes. But as our journey progresses, and we learn from our mistakes, our children will learn too. Personally I have been far from perfect, showing my children my "dark side" more often than I would like. If they do see you act out from anger or ego, talk to them about it. Do not be afraid to apologize and admit you were wrong. Show your children you are working on being a more compassionate, nonjudgmental, loving human being.

Commitment and Service

Commit to what drives you and brings you joy! Commit to parenthood! Commit to showing your children where you stand. Show them that you can be strong enough and brave enough to commit to something you believe in, even though it may not be "following the herd."

Commit to helping others. Commit to protecting the environment. Wherever your passions lie, commit to making a positive contribution and your children will follow your lead.

Bring a sense of service to what you do. Service can occur through your job, volunteering, at home, or just being kind and respectful to others. Being in service is being in the flow of life. We are all here to serve!

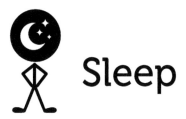

Sleep

Obviously it feels awesome to get a good night's sleep!

Sleep is not a waste of time. Sleep is absolutely essential to wellness. New parents whose infants have their days and nights mixed up can really appreciate the importance of sleep. How wonderful those little naps are during the days you can take them. No matter what else needs to get done, sleep must happen. In fact, we spend one third of our lives sleeping.

During sleep our blood supply and hormones are increased to help with growth and repair of our muscles and organs. Muscles relax and energy is increased in our brains and in our entire bodies. Our blood pressure drops, our breathing slows, and our internal organs rest and rejuvenate for our next waking hours.

Good sleep involves both the Non-Rapid Eye Movement (NREM) and Rapid Eye Movement (REM) states. Not allowing our bodies to get into one or both of these states can lead to significant problems with daytime mental function. Lack of good sleep significantly decreases alertness and memory and increases the risk of injury, especially while driving. It is estimated that more than 100,000 car crashes per year in the U.S. are due to drivers falling asleep behind the wheel.

Getting good sleep may not be that easy. We have all had those nights when we cannot fall asleep or when we wake up and are unable to get back to sleep. Luckily for most of us, this sleep disturbance is not chronic. Unfortunately, chronic insomnia (having sleep disturbance more than three times a week for at least three months) increases the risk of high blood pressure, diabetes, and obesity. Factors that can contribute to insomnia include shift work, light from screened devices, anxiety, depression, or physical discomfort.

Another factor affecting sleep quality is sleep apnea. Sleep apnea occurs when your breathing starts and stops throughout the night decreasing oxygenation to the brain. Signs of sleep apnea include intermittent pauses in breathing which are noticed by others, abrupt awakenings with a feeling of shortness of breath, feeling tired, irritable, or snoring loudly. Uncontrolled sleep apnea may increase weight gain, the risk for heart failure, depression, headaches and attention issues. Talk to your provider if you have chronic sleep issues.

Napping is an important part of the overall sleep pattern in infants and toddlers. There is no specific amount needed, but the overall amount of sleep recommended per day includes naps. When you feel you or your children need a nap, take it! You can actually extend your life expectancy by napping!

Where we sleep is important too. Humans sleep best in a dark, cool and quiet place. It should also be a safe place to sleep. To make sure a child can sleep safely, check that the crib is built to standards and doesn't have anything in or around it that could cause choking or suffocation.

Recommended Amount of Sleep

The following are guidelines issued by the *National Sleep Foundation* for the amount of sleep needed in a 24-hour period for each age group. These numbers include nap time.

○ Newborns (0-3 months)   14–17 hours

○ Infants (4-11 months)   11–14 hours

○ Toddlers (1-2 years)   11–14 hours

○ Preschoolers (3-5 years) 10–13 hours

○ School age (6-13 years)   9–11 hours

○ Teenagers (14-17 years)   8–10 hours

○ Adults (18 and up)   7–9 hours

LEARN MORE ABOUT SLEEP SAFETY:

www.nichd.nih.gov/sts/Pages/default.aspx

www.healthychildren.org

www.sleephealth.org (10 commandments of sleep)

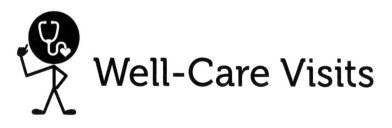

Well-Care Visits

> **Obviously** we want to make sure our children are growing and developing well!

From our baby's first breath to the time they leave the house, it is important to partner with a health care provider who has been trained in pediatrics to help along the way. Well-child visits are a vital tool for keeping our children healthy. During these visits we get to discuss growth and development, preventative care and health history. Well-care visits are also important to screen our children for any physical issues, monitor their vital signs (blood pressure, temperature and pulse), and screen their vision and hearing when appropriate. We can discuss our concerns with an expert in pediatrics about topics such as vaccines, family genetics, development and mental well-being. Building a relationship with a medical provider through well-care visits allows the provider to better serve our children. The American Academy of Pediatrics website has recommendations for well-child visit schedules as well as what to expect from well-checks.

**LEARN MORE FROM THE
AMERICAN ACADEMY OF PEDIATRICS:**

www.aap.org

Immunizations

Of all the topics in pediatric care, vaccination seems to be the one that touches a nerve the most. Vaccinating our children is not only a personal decision but also a community and global decision. On a personal level, we have to decide if the benefits outweigh the risks for our family. From a community standpoint, we have to decide how we will protect those who are more susceptible to diseases, cannot be vaccinated for medical reasons, or do not respond to vaccines.

Many younger parents are not fully aware of the past destruction caused by vaccine-preventable diseases. These parents have never seen, first-hand, a friend or loved one deal with the severe effects of these diseases. Vaccines have helped to reduce the frequency of many diseases and have eliminated some of the diseases altogether. Today we hear about the rare side effects of vaccines just as frequently, or more frequently, than the disability and possible death these maladies cause.

Imagine we are fighting a ghost. Most of us do not see the disease-ghost floating around until it strikes someone we know. Let us become "Ghost Busters" with our prevention-powered immunization packs that blast away vaccine-preventable diseases. When we act as a global community and take the necessary steps to protect ourselves from vaccine-preventable diseases, those diseases disappear completely and we don't have to vaccinate for them anymore. Take smallpox for example. The virus was declared eradicated in 1980 due to mass immunization. We are close to eradicating other vaccine-preventable diseases if we all work together. But if we stop vaccinating too early, that disease will continue to float around and affect those who are susceptible.

Make an informed decision. Don't base this decision on

radical opinions you read online. Base it on statistical evidence. Some of your best resources on vaccines are the people who give them! Ask your health care provider about benefits, risks, and side effects.

LEARN MORE FROM A WONDERFUL BOOK ABOUT THE PSYCHOLOGY OF VACCINE BEHAVIOR:
"On Immunity - An Inoculation" by Eula Biss

Vaccine Effectiveness

Vaccines are considered one of the greatest achievements in medicine. The World Health Organization estimates immunizations save two to three million people per year from vaccine-preventable diseases! Vaccines are typically around 90 percent effective. Studies continue to monitor vaccine effectiveness and recommendations are made based on the results. Unfortunately, these "bugs" we vaccinate against are still floating around and are reappearing in a growing number of outbreaks, in part due to a decline in vaccination rates. The unfortunate realization of these outbreaks is that they involve infants and immune-suppressed individuals who don't have the option to be vaccinated and are at an increased risk of dying from these preventable diseases.

How Vaccines Work

Vaccines work by showing our immune system bits and pieces (antigens) of bacteria and viruses so our bodies will develop a memory (antibodies) that prevent the infection from taking hold during future exposures. The idea is not only to protect us from a possible severe illness, but also to make it less likely we will spread it to others. Vaccines work through personal immunity and also through community immunity (herd immunity). When enough people are vaccinated in a community to make the spread of a disease difficult, both the immune and non-immune populations benefit. To achieve herd immunity there has to be a vaccine rate in that community of 95 percent or greater. That means 95 people out of 100 need to be vaccinated or be immune to that disease. Achieving herd immunity protects everyone in the community from the disease, even those who cannot get the vaccine or don't produce adequate immunity, including newborn babies, the elderly and everyone in-between.

If it were a perfect world, our immune systems would be able to defend against an exposure to almost everything. Unfortunately, there are many factors that play a role in the strength of our immune system, including: internal and external stressors, medications, genetics, age, and nutrition. Even if our immune system could prevent illnesses from all exposures, we still could spread the disease without feeling ill ourselves. We are gambling with our individual health and the health of our loved ones when we don't use the tools our medical and scientific communities have given us.

LEARN MORE ABOUT VACCINE EFFECTIVENESS:

www.vaccines.gov

www.tycho.pitt.edu

www.immunize.org/catg.d/p4037.pdf

www.hhs.gov

www.thescientificparent.org/
vaccines-101-to-much-too-soon

Vaccine Safety

Vaccines are not perfect and do have possible side effects. Most of these side effects are mild and include a localized reaction and a low-grade fever. Severe reactions to vaccines are very rare. In fact, I have seen less than a handful of severe reactions over the past decade. Before vaccines are approved by the FDA they have to undergo years of trials proving their effectiveness and safety. Vaccine safety continues to be monitored closely, even after being introduced to the public, by the Vaccine Adverse Event Reporting System (VAERS). This system is used to gather data on adverse reactions and to advise change in policy if a vaccine is found to be dangerous.

One of the most well-known anti-vaccine papers was published in 1998 by *The Lancet* medical journal. This study was based on only 12 children and proposed a link between the MMR (measles, mumps, rubella) vaccine (specifically the preservative thimerosal*) and autism. The lead investigator of this study lost his medical license after admitting to skewing the data. This study contributed to a widespread fear of a possible link between vaccines and autism, mainly because the scientific community has not been able to identify a specific cause of autism.

More than 20 studies have been published since that infamous 1998 paper and none of them have shown a link between the MMR vaccine and autism. Shortly after the fearful uproar between vaccines and autism, the manufacturers removed thimerosal from almost all of the vaccines even though scientific evidence has proven thimerosal is safe to use in the manufacturing of vaccines.

Another common concern is that we are over-vaccinating infants. Most infants receive 14 vaccines during the first year of their lives, containing 160 immunologic components. In comparison, one bacterium from the environment can have 6,000 immunologic components. As a whole, the stress placed on the immune system is significantly lower with vaccines than it is with natural exposures. As a dad, I will be the first to admit it is not fun watching my children cry during their shots. But until we figure out another way to deliver immunizations, we should think of shots as a loving blessing to protect our children from much more painful diseases.

*Scientific evidence shows us that thimerosal breaks down to **ethyl**mercury, a type of mercury that does not accumulate in the body due to its short half-life and rapid metabolism. **Methyl**mercury, on the other hand, is the type of mercury that can accumulate in our bodies from over-consumption of seafood.

LEARN MORE ABOUT

VACCINE SAFETY AND SIDE EFFECTS:

Vaccine Information Statements (VIS) you should get from your health care provider or at www.hrsa.gov

www.who.int/vaccine_safety/initiative/tools/vaccinfosheets/en/

www.cdc.gov/vaccine safety

Additives in Vaccines

What about the other stuff in vaccines? You know, "all those chemicals and preservatives." Well, that stuff (common additives are formaldehyde and aluminum) helps keep the vaccines safe from contamination, safe to distribute, and makes them more effective. The majority of the additives are only used during the manufacturing of the vaccines. Most are completely removed, or remain only in trace amounts by the time the vaccine is distributed.

Formaldehyde: This additive helps to inactivate viruses like polio and Hepatitis A and toxins like tetanus and diphtheria. By the time the vaccine is shipped out, there is only a trace amount of formaldehyde left (0.02mg per dose). In comparison, a 10-pound baby has 10 times this amount in its blood from normal protein synthesis. That's right, formaldehyde is a natural bi-product of living and is found in all of us!

Aluminum: This is added to induce better immune response (*adjuvant*). It is found naturally in the environment and we are all exposed to aluminum from birth. A breast-fed infant gets 10mg of aluminum from breast milk during the first year of its life. A formula-fed baby gets 120mg of aluminum in its first year. In comparison, vaccines only add around 4mg during the first 12 months of an infant's life.

LEARN MORE ABOUT VACCINE ADDITIVES:
www.publichealth.org
www.cdc.gov/vaccines/vac-gen/additives.htm

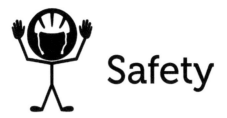

Safety

> **Obviously** your kids should not live in a bubble!

Kids fall a lot. That is part of life. Our bodies are tough and amazing vessels that can take some tumbles. But our bodies are not designed to take the high-speed impact that occurs when a youngster falls off something that propels them faster than nature intended. We will be thankful we took precautions to prevent major injuries when accidents happen. Most safety measures are easy. But what's easy to do is also easy *not* to do. Safety is insurance worth having!

Being safe not only involves wearing *personal protective equipment* (PPE), it also involves body awareness and fitness. Do you want your kids to have a Five Star crash rating? If so, build them strong. Teach them to be aware of their surroundings, and show them it is cool to use PPE.

Since accidents are the number one cause of death from toddlerhood through the teenage years, safety precaution is one of the biggest lifesavers we can implement. The most common accidents that result in death involve motor vehicles. This is no surprise, considering how many cars are on the road and the distractions we all have to deal with in and outside the car. We don't need to teach our kids to fear vehicles, be we do need to teach them to be aware and cautious when around them.

Outside the Car

Street smarts and safety should be taught from the moment children are able to walk. Stop, look both ways, and listen before crossing the street are rules we need to teach our children until the practices become second nature. Using cross walks and making sure drivers see us are basic but critical safety rules. If it is dark out, wear reflective clothing or lights to be more visible to drivers. If children are playing in the street, make sure they watch out for traffic. Make certain they always wear a helmet when riding their bikes, scooters, or anything that makes them go fast. These rules apply while in parking lots, in the street and even in the driveway.

Inside the Car

It is obvious we must follow the laws and regulations for car seats, booster seats, front seat passengers, and seat belt use. As the driver, keep a safe distance from other cars, and don't speed or brake too fast. Keeping our cars maintained will also help reduce accidents. We should respect and care for our cars inside and out and expect our kids to do the same. When driving, focus on driving and nothing else! Avoid using your cell phone, and never text while driving. Avoid driving while sleep-deprived. Follow the *graduated driver licensing program (GDL)* in your state. Stress to your teenager that fatal crashes increase with each teen passenger. Make sure they know that in most fatal crashes involving teenagers, seat belts were not used!

LEARN MORE ABOUT CAR SAFETY:

www.safecar.gov

In the House

It is obvious that we want a safe home for our kids to grow up in. It is fun watching the Addams Family, but I wouldn't want my kids growing up in a house filled with so much potential carnage! So just install padding everywhere and get rid of all chemicals and sharp objects. It's that easy, right? Of course it's not! We have to be practical. We should do our best to re-childproof our homes with the arrival of every new baby. Sometimes it seems like the older sibling's job is to de-childproof our home. It is ok to let minor natural consequences happen. They can be an effective way for our children to learn, as long as there is no permanent bodily damage.

Drowning

Children under five years old have the greatest risk of dying from drowning. It only takes a few inches of water for an infant or young toddler to drown. Prevent drowning by always having an adult watch over children near any kind of water, including the bathtub, pools, rivers, lakes and oceans. Cover or remove all water hazards around the house. Fence off swimming pools and make sure the gate is closed and childproof.

Burns

Children under one year of age have the greatest risk of death from burns. Fire is the most common cause of death, and hot liquids are the most common cause of injury from burns. Make sure your toddler can't reach and spill a pot full of hot or boiling liquid. This includes the coffee pot. Electricity and chemicals are sources of significant burn injuries and death as well. Prevent burns by setting your water heater to 50 degrees Celsius or 120 degrees Fahrenheit or lower. Install smoke detectors in each room of the house. Other potential fire hazards include candles, electric outlets, space heaters, smoking material (cigarettes, pipes, matches, lighters), and dryer machines that are not properly maintained.

Falls

Falls can occur at any age. A baby may fall off the changing table or a toddler may fall down the stairs. Falling is a part of life, but it kills more than 100 kids per day. Prevent falls by installing stair gates and keeping the stairs clear of objects. Install safety windows if your windows are above ground level. Watch your kids closely at playgrounds until you are confident about their climbing abilities. Play at playgrounds with a good landing surface like rubber or updated mulch. Never leave your baby on the changing table or your bed alone, just in case they do a surprise role off of it.

Poisoning

Infants and teenagers are at the greatest risk of dying from ingesting poison. The poison may come from cleaning products, small batteries, personal care products, pesticides, over-the-counter and prescription drugs, and alcohol.

Prevent poisoning by removing all toxic products from your home if you are not going to use them. This can be a hassle because you must dispose of them properly; you can't just throw them away. But it is worth the effort in order to protect your kids and the environment. Store all prescription and non-prescription drugs out of reach, preferably in a locked cabinet.

Store away all of your cleaning products as well, and be aware that even natural products can be toxic. Don't keep it a secret; if youngsters don't know what you are hiding away and the harm those things can cause, their curiosity grows. Show your children what is poisonous and talk to them about the dangers of those poisons.

Make sure you have the local poison control number available and that everyone knows where it is. (I keep mine on the refrigerator door.)

NATIONAL POISON CONTROL:

1-800-222-1222

Firearms

It is obvious you don't want your children to play with a loaded gun in your home or someone else's home. Do not be afraid to ask the adults in homes your children visit frequently if they have firearms and if they keep them locked up. Keep all of your firearms locked up in a safe as well. An uninformed child is a dangerous child. Therefore, teach your children gun safety even if you don't keep guns in your home.

Make sure your children know the difference between a toy gun and a real firearm, and teach them never to touch a real firearm without adult supervision. Nerf guns, water guns, soft air, laser tag, and paintball guns are so common today that you can't expect your children never to aim a gun at someone. Just make sure your children understand that this could prove to be fatal if it is the wrong gun!

Being in the Wrong Place at the Wrong Time

During the school years and through adulthood, some of us have a tendency to be drawn into situations that can put us in harm's way. Hanging around the right people can prevent harm—intentional or unintentional—especially in the teenage years.

Get to know your children's friends and talk to their parents. Teach your children to listen to their gut and to respect themselves enough to prevent peer pressure from controlling their decisions. Remind them that being under the influence of drugs and alcohol can lead to deadly decisions! Let them know that if they are in a situation they need to get out of, they can call you, anytime day or night, and you will come get them, no question asked and no judgment passed.

LEARN MORE ABOUT CHILD SAFETY:
www.safety.org
https://kidshealth.org
www.parents.com/kids/safety/

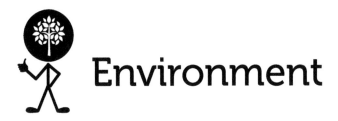

Environment

> **Obviously** we want our children to grow up
> in a healthy environment!

Keeping our internal as well as our external environment clean and healthy is vital for preventing illness and harm. The way we treat the world around us is just as important as the way we treat our bodies. Overwhelming evidence shows that it is difficult to stay healthy if we sicken our environment. Picture a world you want your kids to live in. Imagine the wild, beautiful places you have been or seen. These places won't be around for our children to enjoy if we don't take positive action today!

Airborne Pollution

Smoking

Cigarette smoke contaminates our bodies and the surrounding environment with hundreds of chemicals and carcinogens, all in the name of addiction and that nicotine buzz. Smoking causes more deaths in the U.S. than homicide, car accidents, suicide, alcohol and illegal drugs combined. It is estimated that more than 40 million Americans still smoke! Smoking is the cause of 30 percent of cancers. It is the number one cause of lung cancer and the most important risk factor for head and neck cancers. Up to one out of three deaths from cardiovascular disease is from smoking. One out of five deaths in the United States is from tobacco smoke!

If you currently smoke and plan on becoming a parent, or if you are a parent or caretaker, please stop polluting your body and the environment. Give your kids a fighting chance and don't be a parent or caretaker who smokes.

GREAT RESOURCES TO HELP YOU QUIT SMOKING:

www.quitterscircle.com

www.lung.org

Vaping

Vaping is the act of "smoking" an electronic cigarette. Is it smoking? Not exactly. Is it bad for you? Yes it is! Although no tobacco is involved, it still contains harmful, addicting, cancer-causing chemicals that you breathe into your lungs and out into the environment. The vapor may dissipate faster than smoke but it can still expose others to those chemicals and drugs.

When my boys were younger, I would take them to the skate park to ride their scooters. If one of the older kids started vaping near us, we would have to leave because the smell was so strong! Right now the vaping industry is using "ignorance is bliss" as their marketing tool, stating there are no known deaths from vaping. Of course there aren't, because it hasn't been around long enough to document its deadly effects. We didn't see warning labels on cigarettes until 1966!

Air Pollution

Air pollution affects everyone, including fetuses. Evidence shows that particulate matter given off by planes, trains, and automobiles can cause changes in fetal brain development during the third trimester of pregnancy. These changes increase behavioral problems as well as difficulty focusing when the child grows older.

Air pollution has been linked to pulmonary diseases like asthma. Chronic exposure to air pollution also increases the risk of heart disease, cancer and premature death. Air pollution is also the main contributor to global warming! Along with cars, other major contributors to air pollution include factories, coal-fired power plants, burning wood and raising livestock.

Try to limit your contribution to air pollution by driving less or driving a fuel-efficient car.

Reduce your consumption of food derived from livestock and support clean energy production and the Clean Air Act*.

If you live in or near a large city check your local air quality and if there is a high pollution warning then limit time outside if you have severe asthma or other chronic lung or heart issues.

*Clean Air Act: A federal law put into place in 1970 to help protect human health and the environment from air pollution.

LEARN MORE ABOUT AIR POLLUTION:

www.epa.gov

www.niehs.nih.gov

Planet Earth

Global Warming

Whether you believe the evidence or not, our Earth is warming up. Our planet's temperature is rising ten times faster than normal warming trends. This rapid increase in temperature is correlated with the rapid increase in carbon dioxide in our atmosphere. Carbon dioxide is considered the main greenhouse gas and is produced as a by-product of burning fossil fuels. As these small increases in temperature continue, our environment will continue to change faster than our ability to adapt. These changes include rising sea levels, ocean acidification and increased severe weather patterns. If there were any way to slow global warming, wouldn't you try, for the sake of your children?

LEARN MORE ABOUT GLOBAL WARMING:

https://climate.nasa.gov

Energy

Just like our bodies, we need to fuel our motors and homes with clean energy to keep our environment healthy. We also need to conserve energy so our sources of fuel do not run out. There is more than enough evidence that air pollution from burning fossil fuels is harming our environment and our health. Using renewable energy sources is the way to ease our dependence on fossil fuels. Renewable energy sources include hydropower, geothermal, wind, solar, and biomass. Unlike fossil fuels, renewable energy sources do not directly contribute to greenhouse gases. Unfortunately, only 15 percent of the electricity produced in the United States is from renewable sources. Support the research and development of renewable energy until we can make it affordable and usable.

We need to teach our children how to conserve energy inside and outside the home. Education is a powerful tool in saving our earth. We should teach our kids to turn off lights when not using them. Show them how to use a programmable thermostat. Encourage them to avoid wasting hot water. Children who learn to be responsible with energy conservation and recycling will find it natural to live this way as adults.

LEARN MORE ABOUT CLEAN ENERGY:

www.nrdc.org

www.nrel.gov

Water

There is a limited amount of fresh water on this planet. We know that 70 percent of the earth is covered by water, but the majority of it is undrinkable and is being polluted at alarming rates. A lack of clean water sources is one of the biggest global health problems we face. We should teach our children how to conserve water by turning off the faucet when brushing their teeth and limiting how long they shower and how many baths they take. Use newer, more water efficient showerheads, faucets, dishwashers, and washing machines, and turn off the garden hose when not in use. We should show them how to conserve water outside the home as well with xeriscaping or good lawn-watering practices if lawn watering is absolutely necessary. Support research and development of water conservation and clean water sources.

LEARN MORE ABOUT CLEAN WATER:

www.nature.org

www.greenfacts.org

Recycling

In the United States, we only recycle about 20 percent of our waste, despite the fact that recycling keeps pollutants from going into our landfills and oceans. Recycling helps conserve fresh water that would otherwise be used in the manufacturing of raw materials. Recycling also helps preserve other natural resources including fossil fuels and our forests. Recycling reduces air pollution created by manufacturing raw materials. In fact, recycling paper products produces 70 percent less air pollution compared to making paper from raw material.

To help increase recycling, buy products that can be recycled or are made from recycled material. Sign up for the local recycling program offered by your garbage collector. Place recycling bins where you won't forget to use them. Teach your kids which packaging and materials can be recycled and show them how easy it is to do it correctly. A few ideas for recycling outside the home include: recycling grass clippings back into the soil by using a mulching lawn mower, composting, and using the recycle bins at stores and restaurants.

Agriculture

Raising livestock can have a negative impact on the environment if not done responsibly. Ranching requires a large amount of land and fresh water. In fact, approximately 30 percent of the earth's land is used to grow food for livestock instead of humans! Raising livestock requires the use of large amounts of chemical pollutants including herbicides, pesticides, and antibiotics, none of which are good for us or the earth. Support earth-friendly practices by consuming organic and free range animal and plant products. Buy locally grown produce to reduce the energy and resources needed to get food to our tables. We should try growing our own gardens or use a community garden to help teach your kids where food comes from and have them participate in the magic of growing their own food. My boys have helped with our vegetable garden since before they could walk. We'd plop them down in the middle of the garden and let them play in the dirt while we worked around them. This early and consistent exposure to growing their own food has helped make them less picky eaters. It also makes them appreciate the value and importance of good healthy food.

LEARN MORE ABOUT AGRICULTURAL PRACTICES:

www.nrdc.org

www.ewg.org

www.fao.org

Those Other Creatures

All living creatures are part of an intricate web of life where everyone is affected even if one creature becomes extinct. As humans, we should make it a goal not to make a species disappear due to our actions. We need to teach our kids about all the wonderful, diverse, living creatures with whom we share Mother Earth.

When we get our children out of the house and into nature to observe our critter friends and their habitats, we teach them to respect both the animal and plant kingdoms. We can also visit a zoo and support organizations that help protect wildlife.

ORGANIZATIONS YOU COULD HELP SUPPORT:
www.worldwildlife.org
www.nwf.org
www.everythingconnects.org

Deforestation

Rainforests are one of earth's treasures because they:

○ Produce 20 percent of the planet's oxygen.

○ Help keep water vapor in the air and slow global warming.

○ Are the home for 70 percent of all the plant and animal species on earth.

○ Are the source of hundreds of medical remedies and herbs that are still to be discovered.

Unfortunately, the rainforests on our planet are being destroyed at an alarming rate. In fact, if we continue at the current rate of destruction, all rainforests could be eliminated in only 100 years. That means our grandchildren and their great-grandchildren will never get to experience the amazing gifts of the rainforest.

However, we can all do our part to protect the rainforests! We can support companies with "zero deforestation" policies or are a part of the *Forest Stewardship Council*. We can buy recycled or certified sustainable wood if we have to buy wood. One of the biggest reasons for deforestation is clearing land for agriculture. Less demand for cow products like beef and dairy means less need for deforestation. We can try to limit our intake of beef and dairy and purchase those products from local sources when necessary.

Caring for our planet is such an important part of wellness. We all have the power to be a positive force for Mother Earth.

TO LEARN MORE ABOUT RAINFORESTS:

www.rainforest-alliance.org

https://rainforests.mongobay.com

www.nationalgeographic.com/environment/ habitats/rain-forests/

MY OBVIOUS PARENTING PLAN

Part Two

The Stages of Development

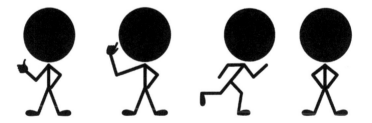

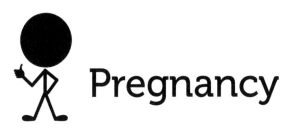

Pregnancy

> **Obviously** pregnancy can be one of the most precious gifts you will ever receive!

Amazing changes occur during the first few weeks of pregnancy. Imagine, by four weeks after conception your baby's heart will begin to beat! Unfortunately, you often don't know you are pregnant until after those first heartbeats. Pregnancy tests can tell you sooner, but most likely you won't know to take a test because you won't suspect pregnancy until you miss your first period. The majority of birth defects develop during the first trimester of pregnancy.

If you want to prevent or decrease the risk of birth defects, start treating your body correctly before you ever get pregnant. Because abstinence is the only 100 percent guaranteed form of birth control, if you are having intercourse with the opposite sex then the potential to get pregnant is there.

Taking care of yourself means you are taking care of a possible new life. Avoid alcohol, tobacco, marijuana or any other illegal drugs. If you are trying to get pregnant, check with your doctor if you are taking any medications or herbs. Make sure you are protected from infections that can cause birth defects like rubella and chickenpox through immunizations or antibody testing. If you have diabetes make sure it is controlled.

Being obese during pregnancy is also a risk factor for birth defects so work to achieve a healthy weight prior to pregnancy.

Potential fathers need to do the same. Don't gain that "sympathy weight." Start or continue those healthy habits that keep your body strong and healthy. It is important to be in a stable relationship or have some type of support system if you plan on getting pregnant. Having a supportive and involved partner for your children significantly improves their chances of succeeding in life. Work on strengthening your relationship before and during pregnancy; your children will thank you.

Nutrition During Pregnancy

Obviously you want to feed yourself and the little one growing inside you healthy foods.

It is critical to the baby's health that the mother be healthy, so adopting a healthy lifestyle long before getting pregnant is ideal. Nutritionally, a healthy lifestyle includes a wide variety of fruits, vegetables, whole grains and protein sources.

Here are some specific nutrients you need to think about when you arc pregnant. (Make sure you discuss the specifics with your health care provider).

Folic Acid (folate)

To reduce neural-tube defects you should be getting approximately 800 micrograms of folic acid per day via green leafy vegetables, citrus fruits, beans, and a prenatal vitamin if necessary.

Another important nutrient that helps prevent neural-tube defects is choline. You should get around 450mg of choline per day via seeds, soybeans, collard greens, shrimp, eggs, and poultry.

Iron

Your body uses iron to make hemoglobin. Hemoglobin is in your red blood cells and is used to carry oxygen to all the tissues in your body. During pregnancy your need for iron is doubled due to your increased blood volume. You should get around 27mg of iron per day via nuts, dried fruit, collard greens, meats, and fortified cereals. Heme iron from animal sources has been shown to absorb better than non-heme iron from plant sources. You can enhance the absorption of iron from non-animal sources by combining it with a vitamin C supplement or vitamin C-rich foods including citrus fruits and vegetables like bell peppers, kale and broccoli.

B-Vitamins

Besides folic acid there are seven other B-vitamins that are important during pregnancy. B-vitamins are important due to their ability to help your body use and produce energy. Good sources of these vitamins include fruits, vegetables and beans. Vitamin B-12 is the only B-vitamin that is difficult to find in plant products so if you are a vegetarian or vegan, you should consider taking a supplement. Most prenatal vitamins include all of these B-vitamins.

Healthy Fats

Fats are essential for the development of our nervous systems and cell development. Eat a diet rich in unsaturated fats (poly- and mono-unsaturated) from fish, nuts, oils, and soybeans. Limit saturated fats, especially from red meats, and completely avoid trans-fats like partially hydrogenated oils (found in many packaged foods).

Protein

During pregnancy your body has an increased need for proteins. Proteins are the building blocks for growth and development. You should be consuming around 60-70 grams of protein per day through nuts, seeds, beans, tofu, whole grains, dairy, and meats.

Hydration

You should be drinking around 10 cups, or two and a half liters of water per day, to make up for the increased blood volume caused by pregnancy. Most of your water intake should happen earlier in the day to avoid interrupting your sleep with trips to the bathroom throughout the night.

Calories

You should be eating around 300 more calories per day during your second trimester, and around 450 more calories per day during your third trimester. This increase in calories should allow you to gain around 25–35 pounds during pregnancy, unless you are already over or under your ideal body weight for your age and height. Being obese could increase your risk of having a stillbirth by 25 percent! Being underweight can slightly increase the risk of having a premature birth or underweight baby. Talk to your provider about your specific weight goals during pregnancy.

Things to Limit or Avoid While You are Pregnant

You should limit your **caffeine** intake to less than 200mg, or 2 cups of coffee per day, to decrease the risk of miscarriage and low birth weight. You should limit preformed (active form) vitamin A to less than 2,500 IU per day to avoid increased risk of birth defects. Concentrated sources of preformed vitamin A come from vitamins, certain medications, eggs, milk, and certain seafood including cod, salmon, and oysters. Vitamin A from beta-carotene (not preformed) has not been found to cause birth defects.

Try to limit **fish that is high in methylmercury.** These include swordfish, shark, king mackerel, tilefish, tuna, shrimp, salmon and cod. Avoid foods that carry a higher risk of food-borne illness from bacterial contamination including unpasteurized dairy, uncooked meats, uncooked eggs, and fresh sprouts. Avoid alcohol because there is no safe amount during any trimester of pregnancy.

Exercise During Pregnancy

Obviously you want to move more
than the baby in your belly!

You should definitely exercise during pregnancy unless your health care provider suggests different. Benefits of exercising during pregnancy include improved sleep, muscle tone, strength, and endurance, which will help you prepare for labor and delivery. Being fit will also help you with recovery from delivery so you can get back to normalcy as soon as possible. Exercising can also help reduce the stress on your pelvis and lower back from the physical imbalances of pregnancy.

Safe Exercises

Safe exercises during pregnancy include walking, swimming, cycling, aerobics and running. Keep in mind that you can get over-heated more easily when pregnant. You should avoid any activity that increases the risk of falling. These activities may include skiing, horseback riding and contact sports. You should also avoid scuba diving due to its inherent risks. Try to avoid exercises on your back after the first trimester because the weight of your uterus could put pressure on a large vein in your abdomen, possibly affecting blood flow to your brain and the baby. There are no specific heart rate goals during pregnancy but you should be able to have a conversation while exercising and if you can't, slow down.

Spirituality During Pregnancy

Obviously you are truly connected
with the child in your belly!

If you are thinking about becoming pregnant or you already are, then this is a perfect time to reflect on how amazing you are! The ability to create another human being inside you is incredible. Your body's ability to adapt to and nurture the rapidly growing baby is one of the wonders of nature. When you fill yourself with positive thoughts and loving energy you are automatically giving that love and optimism to your baby. If you feel the joy of loving yourself, so will the one(s) inside of you. This love and respect will multiply if shared with your partner and those you are close to.

Oneness

You are truly never alone, especially when you are pregnant. There is an undeniable physical and spiritual oneness with you and your baby. What a special gift! The oneness doesn't stop there. Continue to realize the oneness in your community and especially with your partner. Take advantage of "expecting" and go to pregnancy related classes, especially when you are pregnant with your first child.

Gratitude

What an amazing gift you have or will receive. Be grateful for every day you are pregnant, even on those rough days. Being thankful for every step during the journey of pregnancy is far better than worrying about and focusing on the discomforts.

Optimism

Positive thoughts turn into positive energy that flows between you and the one growing inside you. On the other hand, stressful thoughts may cause a physical stress response that can include increased heart rate, increased blood pressure and the release of stress hormones that can affect your baby. Go with the flow and let the child inside you peacefully grow!

Sleep During Pregnancy

Obviously you need lots of sleep to support you and your growing baby.

When you are pregnant, you are snoozing for two. A chronic lack of sleep (less than six hours a night) can increase the risk of having a cesarean (c-section) and a longer labor. Get used to taking naps when you can; you will need this skill when your baby arrives. You should sleep on your side, preferably your left side. Use extra pillows placed in supportive positions like between your arms and thighs. If you have a history of sleep apnea, make sure it is controlled because sleep apnea could increase the risk of high blood pressure and preeclampsia.

Factors that can possibly decrease a good night's sleep include increased urinary frequency, heartburn, sinus congestion and restless leg syndrome. Talk to your provider if you feel any of these are affecting your sleep.

Well-Care: Prenatal Visits

Obviously you want to make sure you stay healthy during pregnancy!

Prenatal visits are very important for keeping track of how you and your growing baby are doing. From vital signs and measurements to ultrasounds, keeping up to date on how things are going can improve the outcome of your pregnancy.

The first prenatal visit is usually around the eighth week of pregnancy and includes measurements of your blood pressure, height, weight, a physical exam including a pelvic exam, and confirming your pregnancy via urine or blood. Your provider may also check for bacteria in your urine, check your blood for your blood type (Rh factor), get a complete blood count, and check for infections including Hepatitis B, HIV, syphilis, and rubella.

The frequency of your prenatal visits will be determined by your provider, but they generally include monthly visits under 28 weeks of pregnancy, biweekly visits from 28 to 36 weeks, and weekly visits after your 36th week of pregnancy.

Discuss with your provider the vaccines you need to have before pregnancy and which ones are safe during pregnancy. If you are not fully vaccinated you can get most vaccines when you are pregnant. Exceptions are the live vaccines, including MMR (measles, mumps, rubela), Varivax (chicken pox), and FluMist. It is now recommended that you receive a Tdap (tetanus/whooping cough) shot and flu shot during every pregnancy. Some of the antibodies your body produces after receiving a vaccine can pass through to your baby, protecting them when born. This is a good time to learn about childhood vaccines and their recommended schedule.

Safety During Pregnancy

Obviously you want to keep that growing baby safe!

Not only do you need to think about your own safety and the safety of your growing baby, but this is also the time to start taking safety measures for when they are living outside the womb. Near the end of pregnancy you will need to purchase a car seat and properly install it in your car. If you are going to use a crib, check for recalls because some older cribs can become a suffocation or entrapment hazard due to faulty dropside mechanics and other problems.

Other safety items to consider before your baby arrives:

○ A changing table with a safety strap

○ Baby gates for top and/or bottom of the stairs

○ Child-proof hooks for cabinets and drawers

○ Child-proof door handles

○ Furniture anchors

○ Smoke detectors and carbon monoxide detectors

○ Electrical outlet covers

LEARN MORE ABOUT CAR SEATS & CRIB RECALLS:

www.safecar.gov

www.parents.com recall page

Environment During Pregnancy

Obviously your baby is going to live on this earth with you, so treat it with respect!

If you are not already in the habit of saving energy, recycling and conserving water, now is the time to get into those habits. Use reusable water bottles, recycle when you can, and don't let water run unless it is being used. A bonus is that these steps will cut down on your energy bill! Turn lights off, use LED lights, have a programmable thermostat, unplug small appliances, and have an efficient water heater.

In an ideal world, we would all live close to the places where we go to the most in order to reduce the amount of time we spend in the car. This isn't always possible or practical; my wife and I are guilty of driving too much! We try to balance this and reduce our carbon footprint by combining errands and riding our bikes whenever possible.

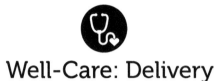

Well-Care: Delivery

Obviously you want the birth of your child to be a smooth and safe experience for everyone.

Delivery of your newborn may not go as planned. Keep an open mind for whatever delivery type is needed to keep you and your baby safe. It may be helpful to write a spiritual birthing plan to affirm your gratefulness for having a healthy delivery, no matter what type of delivery it is. There are two types of delivery:

Vaginal

If possible, a vaginal delivery is preferred. This is the way your baby is designed to come out! There are several benefits of vaginal delivery. First, you are obviously less likely to need a surgical procedure. Second, vaginal delivery usually results in a faster recovery for the mom and baby. And finally, vaginal delivery will expose your baby to natural vaginal flora (bacteria) to help colonize their intestines and prime their immune systems.

A **natural delivery** means you are not using any IV medication, including an epidural*. The benefits of a natural delivery include a quicker recovery time and improved initial breastfeeding and bonding with your child. Sedative painkillers and other medication can slow the interactions between the two of you. Natural deliveries have less possible complications from medications and epidurals, as well as less need for urinary catheterization.

***epidural:** injection of local pain medication outside the dura mater of the spinal cord to produce loss of sensation of the pelvis and legs.

C-Section

Having a cesarean section can save your life and the life of your child. However, studies show there are too many being done electively. C-sections are surgical procedures, so they have the same risks as other surgeries. You will most likely be at the hospital longer due to your recovery. Some babies born by c-section may have a more difficult time breastfeeding initially. It also may take longer for your baby to adjust to being outside the womb due to medication exposure and less immediate contact with you. But if your baby is in distress and the doctor advises a c-section, it is important to understand this decision and feel good about it.

Cutting the Cord

There is no universally recommended time to clamp and cut the umbilical cord, but the World Health Organization recommends waiting at least one minute post delivery. Delaying cord clamping can potentially improve your baby's hemoglobin level and blood volume by about half a cup, and potentially improve their cognitive ability as a toddler. Delaying cord cutting may also decrease the need for iron supplementation for exclusively breastfed infants. Talk to your delivery team about their cord cutting policy.

Washing Your Baby Off

Most hospitals bathe an infant soon after birth but just like cord cutting, there is a growing trend to delay the bath. Delaying the first bath may help keep your child protected by not immediately washing off their natural vernix* coating. Delaying the bath could also help keep their body temperature stable by avoiding temperature fluctuations from water exposure and evaporation. It also allows more immediate skin-to-skin contact with mother. The World Health Organization recommends not washing your baby off until they are at least 24 hours old. Speak to your delivery team about their bathing policy.

*vernix: a protective coating consisting of skin oils and dead skin cells on a newborn.

MY OBVIOUS PARENTING PLAN
for Pregnancy

Notes

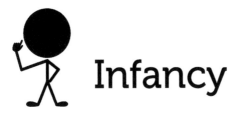 Infancy

> **Obviously** you want to start your baby's journey
> outside the womb on the right foot!

Shortly after delivery your baby will be measured, Apgar scores* will be assessed, and a Vitamin K shot will be given along with antibiotic eye ointment. If you are planning on breastfeeding, try to have your baby latch on as soon as possible to improve the likelihood of breastfeeding success.

***Apgar score:** Apgar is an acronym for Appearance, Pulse, Grimace, Activity, Respiration. This is a quick test given at one minute and five minutes after birth to monitor your baby's transition outside the womb.

Vitamin K

The vitamin K shot is given after delivery to decrease the risk of your baby having a brain bleed. Less than one percent of babies have Vitamin K Deficiency Bleeding, but one out of five that have the deficiency will die! There is no significant evidence of any short-term or long-term side effects of this shot, and it could save your baby's life.

Antibiotic Eye Ointment

Antibiotic eye ointment (usually erythromycin) is applied to prevent a bacterial eye infection (i.e., Chlamydia, Gonorrhea, and E. coli) that could lead to blindness. A rare side effect of the ointment is a local allergic reaction. Eye ointment may not be necessary right away, and may not be necessary at all if you had a c-section.

Critical Congenital Heart Disease (CCHD) Screen

This simple pulse oxygen test is done 24 hours after birth and can help pick up heart defects that, if detected early, can have a better outcome.

Newborn Screen

The Newborn Screen is performed within a few days of birth and tests up to 50 genetic, metabolic, and endocrine disorders that, if caught early, have a better outcome. This test is repeated in 10-14 days to make sure later developing markers are caught.

LEARN MORE ABOUT NEWBORN SCREENING:

www.savebabies.org

Hearing Screening

All newborns should have a hearing screening done. It is not uncommon for babies to fail their first screening due to residual vernix in the ear canals. If they fail the first screening, a repeat screen will be conducted prior to discharge, or you may need to return to the hospital for this second screening. Just like with the newborn screen, earlier detection of hearing loss has a better outcome.

Nutrition During Infancy

> **Obviously** you want to give your growing
> infant optimal nutrition.

Nutrition for your baby during the first few months of life are simple: breast milk, some type of formula, or both.

Breastfeeding

Breastfeeding is what nature intended and nature knows best! Breast milk is considered the optimal nutrition for your infant during their first four to six months of life or longer. Here are just a few benefits of breastfeeding:

○ Helps mom lose weight

○ On-demand supply

○ Perfectly formulated for your child

○ Already warmed up

○ Provides great bonding with mom

○ Contains natural probiotics

○ The taste and nutrients from mom's diet decreases pickiness and allergies later in life

○ Environmentally friendly (less packaging and processing!)

○ Less chance of constipation for your baby

○ Less stinky diapers compared to formula

○ Decreases risk of diabetes and childhood leukemia

○ Possible increased IQ for child

○ It's free!

New mothers, be patient! It may take three to five days for breast milk to come in, but your colostrum* comes in immediately, and although there is only a small amount, it is liquid gold. Newborns do not require a lot of volume the first few days. It can be normal for your baby to lose up to 10 percent of their weight during the first four to five days.

The mechanics of breastfeeding are different than sucking on a bottle or pacifier. A general rule is to avoid using a bottle until at least two weeks after birth to decrease nipple confusion. Pacifier use in the first few days can affect breastfeeding as well, so if you are using a bottle or pacifier and it is affecting your baby's latch, stop if possible until they are a few weeks older.

If you are going to breastfeed make sure you are eating a well-rounded diet full of fruits and vegetables and whole grains. The more diverse a mother's diet is, the less likely allergies and pickiness will develop in toddlerhood. Make sure you are eating plenty of protein through plant or animal sources. Limit your caffeine to less than the equivalent of three cups of coffee per day. If you drink alcohol, limit it to one drink per day and wait at least two hours after your drink to breastfeed. Continue to limit high mercury fish. Prescriptions should always be checked by the prescriber to see if they are safe to take while breastfeeding. And of course, don't do recreational drugs.

*__Colostrum:__ Rich in immune protective substances and proteins, colostrum is the secretion produced by mammary glands of mammals late in pregnancy and through the first few days after birth before true breast milk comes in.

Donor Breast Milk

If you get breast milk from a breast milk bank, it will be pasteurized to decrease the risk of bacterial contamination. Pasteurization has been shown to decrease some active immune components and some vitamins and enzymes in the breast milk, but it still contains the majority of Mother Nature's recipe. Milk from milk-sharing sites is not usually regulated. This could increase the risk of the donor milk having an abnormal bacterial load that could make your baby sick. Be very careful getting breast milk from someone you don't know!

Storage of Breast Milk

Breast milk should be safe for four days in the fridge, six months in a freezer, and nine months in a deep freezer. You should use it within 24 hours after it is thawed, and one hour after feeding with it if there is some left. Never water breast milk down unless directed by a provider. Never microwave breast milk or formula, and always test the temperature of breast milk or formula on yourself first, preferably on a sensitive part of your body such as the underside of your wrist.

Formula

Sometimes breastfeeding doesn't work out. This doesn't make you a bad mom and is no cause for guilt. When the decision is made to use the bottle exclusively, don't look back! Breastfeeding was a struggle for my fair-skinned wife with both of our boys. She tried everything, pumped day and night, and breastfed as long as she could. She loved the idea of breastfeeding, but the act truly stressed her out. When she finally switched to formula, she was a much happier mom (and wife)! There have been millions of people in the past 50 years nourished by formula who are wonderfully healthy!

It can be overwhelming to choose a formula for your infant. For the most part you will have to try one and if your baby is not doing well on it, switch to a different one. Formulas are highly regulated by the Federal Drug Administration (FDA), so even generic formulas are safe. I recommend starting with a partially broken down (hydrolyzed) whey-based protein formula due to evidence that it can help decrease food allergies, eczema, and constipation. Almost every major formula brand makes a partially broken down protein formula.

If your baby is having issues with a cow milk formula, then try a soy-based formula or a more fully broken down formula. There are also specialized formulas that need a prescription, so ask your provider for details. There is no solid evidence that soy formulas have any more complications then cow milk formulas, so if you would like to try a soy-based formula, go for it. Using an organic formula is wonderful, but there are fewer options for organic formulas and they are more expensive. The use of premixed formulas versus powder is going to be up to you, but occasionally I see babies do better on premixed formulas.

Solids

You can start feeding your infant solids at four to six months of age. Make sure your baby can hold their head up, sit upright, and weighs approximately twice their birth weight. Most babies will either be reaching for your food or opening their mouths and leaning into your food when they are ready to start solids.

There are no specific rules regarding which solid food to start with, but you do want to avoid whole milk and raw honey until your baby is around 12 months old. Whole cow milk has a large protein that can be irritating to a maturing digestive system. Raw honey may contain botulism, a bacterium that releases a toxin which causes paralysis in some infants with less mature digestive systems or compromised immune systems. You should also limit the amount of rice cereal due to rice's naturally higher concentration of arsenic.

Try to introduce a variety of foods before one year of age. This includes the more allergenic foods, like nut butters, as they can decrease the development of food allergies. You can start with purees, finger foods or a combination of both.

Be careful to avoid foods that can be a choking hazard including any food that is round, hard to dissolve in the mouth, or could block the airway. Your baby may gag on solids until they are used to swallowing something other than liquids.

Introduce new foods one at a time, every three to four days, to avoid confusion if they do have a reaction. Increase the amount of feedings from once a day to two or three times a day after they grow more comfortable with eating solids. This usually occurs around six to nine months of age.

Eat with your baby, include them at family meals, and share your food with them as tolerated.

Exercising with Infants

> **Obviously** you want your baby to use his
> or her body to play and have fun!

Raising an infant is already taxing with the constant lack of sleep and everyday parenting duties. It's no wonder that exercise is one of the last things on the minds of new parents. Keeping up with an infant can be enough movement, but make sure you are getting your heart rate up.

If you make movement a habit when your children are infants, you are better able to keep up with them when they are older. Take them in baby carriers when you go on walks or hikes as much as possible. Get them used to being outdoors and moving, even though they are not moving much themselves. This will help ward off the cabin fever I often see in parents during the first six months of their parenting.

You can start using a jogging stroller when your baby is around six months old or sturdy enough to sit upright. Look for jogging strollers and bike trailers that allow the seat to recline. Most experts advise not using a bike trailer until babies are at least 12 months old due to possible injuries from crashing.

Play with your baby! They are more likely to move when you play with them. I know they are wonderful to hold, but set them down and allow them freedom to explore. Give them toys to reach for. Help them to stand before four months old to give them that feeling of pressure on their legs. At around six to nine months old, start having them play while standing and leaning or holding onto something.

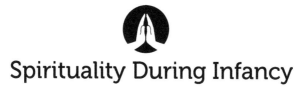

Spirituality During Infancy

It is **obvious** your baby is closer to "the source."

Early parenthood is a perfect time to bring yourself back to the simplicity of life. Follow your infant's lead in being non-judgmental, loving and honest. Enjoy the simplicity of a touch, taking a nap, and eating to live, rather than eating to fill emotional voids. We can see what it is like to be closer to our spiritual source when we watch a baby. They have not developed opinions or an ego. Their minds are not tainted with memories, behaviors or learned emotions. They are pure spiritual beings starting the physical human journey. Infants are not worried about the past or future like most adults are. Look into your baby's eyes and see the present moment!

Even though they are pure beings, babies must adjust to the world outside the womb. They need to figure out their bodies and the physical signals their bodies send. This can be a struggle for some. Be there to help comfort and support them when they cry because of an uncomfortable feeling. Remember their actions are never for spite. Try to work as a parental team and as part of a larger community when raising an infant. This will help you take care of yourself and expose your baby to many loving hands.

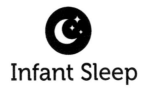

Infant Sleep

> **Obviously** you want your baby
> to "sleep like a baby."

Sometimes you don't appreciate how nice it is to sleep through the night until you have a baby. If you have never been someone who naps, this is a time to learn to enjoy naps. Newborns can sleep up to 18 hours a day, mostly in the form of multiple short naps. Infants and toddlers also spend more time than adults in REM sleep (Rapid Eye Movement sleep, characterized by dreaming and body movement), which means they are light sleepers.

Do not stress out about not sleeping through the night. It can take a few months for your little ones to figure out their sleep cycle outside the womb. If you think about it, their nervous systems have to adjust to an onslaught of stimuli and then figure out how to relax enough to fall asleep. This can be a difficult adjustment for some. You use your touch to soothe them from the very beginning, so when you start having them settle to sleep without your constant touch, understand why they cry. Be patient with yourself and with your baby.

To help your baby sleep better at night:

○ Keep them active during the day.

○ Keep the atmosphere light and energetic during the day, but if your baby is getting fussy, calm them down and allow them to sleep. You do not want to over-stimulate them.

○ Start a bedtime routine after a few weeks. This may include a bath, a bedtime story, singing, music, massage, or any other soothing habit.

○ Try not to have them fall asleep in your arms. Put them down in their own crib or cradle while they are dozing off, but not asleep.

○ Know that co-sleeping can increase SIDS (Sudden Infant Death Syndrome) and co-sleeping babies tend to wake more often. (See page 101 for more on SIDS)

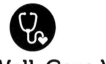

Infant Well-Care Visits

It is **obvious** you want to make sure
your baby is developing well.

Well-child visits during infancy are a great time to let your pediatric provider get to know you. It is important to build a trusting relationship with your baby's health care provider.

Your baby's first check-up should occur two to five days after delivery. During this first visit, your provider will check for jaundice, make sure feedings are going well, make sure your baby has not lost too much weight, and address any concerns that have developed at home.

The next visit is usually around two weeks after birth, followed by well-checks at two, four, six, nine, and twelve months. During these visits, growth and development will be assessed, as will eating, sleeping, and voiding habits. Vaccines will be recommended and given if appropriate, and any concerns will hopefully be addressed.

Vaccines

The first recommended vaccine for your baby will be shortly after delivery. It is recommended to start the Hepatitis B vaccine around birth to decrease the risk of chronic complications from this virus that may not be picked up during prenatal screenings. Studies have proven this vaccine to be safe and effective.

The first "set" of vaccines are recommended at the two-month well-child check. Vaccines are started early not because your baby's immune system is weak, but because some infants can develop serious complications from contracting vaccine-preventable diseases. Think of vaccines as teachers to your child's immune system. They teach our immune systems how to recognize a potential disease and prevent that virus or bacteria from being able to overwhelm our bodies. This is not unlike teaching your kids seatbelt use and street safety to prevent injury or death from a car crash. We cannot get rid of all the bacteria and viruses in the world, just like we will not get rid of cars any time soon. Talk to your provider about vaccines as soon as possible.

Inform yourself about vaccines by reading the Vaccine Information Statement for each vaccine. These can be found at your pediatrician's office or online at www.cdc.gov.

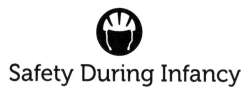

Safety During Infancy

Obviously you want to keep your baby out of harm's way while letting them explore this new and exciting world!

Car Seats

Before taking your baby home from the hospital or birthing center you should have a rear-facing car seat properly installed. Most fire stations have a trained car seat inspector that can help you install it properly. Your baby's car seat should be positioned in the middle of the back seat and rear facing if possible.

Home Safety

Once your infant starts moving they can get into trouble. Even a two-month old can do an unexpected roll while on the changing table, so do not leave them alone anywhere they could possibly fall off. At around six months old, infants can start moving from point A to point B. Point B is often something that could harm them, like a cord to chew on, stairs to fall down, or a dog that doesn't like to be bothered. For the most part, infants instinctively know their limits, but don't trust that. Childproof your home from the ground up. Curiosity is how babies learn but it can also get them into trouble. Put safety latches and locks on cabinets and drawers. Be very careful about where you store button batteries. Not only are they a choking hazard but they are small enough to be swallowed and their acid is toxic! Also be cautious about potential burns from scalding water, fireplaces, and vaporizers.

Sudden Infant Death Syndrome (SIDS) or Sudden Unexplained Infant Death (SUID)

SIDS is the unexplained death of an otherwise healthy baby, usually while asleep. Scientists believe it could be linked to an abnormal brain development that alters the carbon dioxide sensors responsible for signaling the body to move out of an asphyxiating position. Over 3,000 infants per year in the United States die of SIDS. Risk factors for SIDS include low birth weight, respiratory infections, sleeping on the belly, sleeping on soft surfaces, second hand smoke, prematurity, and maternal use of alcohol. Have your baby sleep on their back on a firm surface with no suffocating material around. There is evidence that pacifier use and a fan running in the room can decrease SIDS as well.

Crib Safety

Make sure there are no gaps greater than the width of two fingers between the mattress and railing. Don't place cords near the crib that your baby could reach and possibly wrap around their neck. Avoid using a crib over ten years old, one that has been recalled, or a crib with a drop-side.

Water Safety

Never leave your infant alone in a bath! Babies can drown in only a few inches of water. Make sure there are no unattended containers of water your baby can fit in when they are able to move themselves around the house, even scooting and crawling. Close toilet lids, empty baby pools when not using them, and install alarms and safety covers on hot tubs and pools. It is important to learn infant CPR as well.

Environment During Infancy

Obviously you do not want to stress Mother Earth with all the crap it takes to raise a baby!

This is a time to continue environmentally friendly habits, and start new ones. Continue to get out into nature with your little one. Let them feel cool and warm days, the breeze, even rain and snow (as long as you dress them appropriately). Start using more natural cleaners that are safer for your family and the environment. Conserve water whenever possible. It is nice to fill up a small infant bathtub instead of the whole tub. Conserve energy by turning off lights and the TV. Letting your baby watch TV could be harmful anyway*.

*Studies have shown allowing children under 18 months old to view screens for an extended period of time can affect language development and reading skills. It can also disrupt their sleep and cause attention issues.

Diapers

One of the most obvious environmental decisions during your child's first few years is what kind of diapers to use. No matter what type of diaper parents choose, they quickly become diaper-changing professionals! There are pros and cons for both cloth and disposable diapers.

At first glance it would seem that cloth diapers are more earth-friendly because they are not made of synthetic materials, including petroleum products. Cloth diapers do not fill our landfills. Newer cloth diapers also have less washable material so fewer resources are used to clean them, and there are several different types to fit your baby's needs. They are manufactured using fewer raw materials including trees. But cloth diapers have their own dirty secrets. Cloth diapers are made from cotton, which happens to be one of the most water and pesticide demanding crops we grow. Cloth diapers are also highly refined and take large amounts of energy and water to make and take care of.

Disposable diapers are slightly easier to use because you simply throw them away when they are dirty. Plus, disposable diapers seem to fit better on newborns. Unfortunately, we fill our landfills with 3.4 million tons of diapers each year. That's more than 20 billion disposable diapers, and they take hundreds of years to decompose! Some disposable diaper companies are making their diapers more earth-friendly with less waste material and more biodegradable materials that are renewable.

No matter which you choose, try to use a company that is making a true effort to develop more earth-friendly products. Some infants have fewer diaper rashes with one or the other, or one brand fits better than another. In these cases, your decision is easy: choose the diaper that is most comfortable for your baby.

MY OBVIOUS PARENTING PLAN
for Infancy

Notes

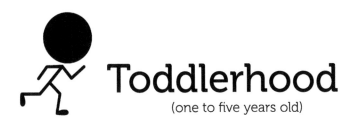

Toddlerhood
(one to five years old)

> It is **obvious** that raising a toddler can get a little crazy.
> This is a great time to have fun with your crazy kid.

The toddler years can certainly be a little crazy. Toddlers will say and do things that will surprise you, embarrass you, and make you laugh and cry at the same time.

As a parent, this is a great time to improve your multitasking skills but at the same time stay centered. When my boys were toddlers, I personally had to re-evaluate those "boundaries" I had set for my family because they were pushed every single day. This is a time to let go of our preconceived notions that our toddlers should know all the rules and follow them. Rather, it's a time to let down our guard and get a little crazy with them. I promise it will make this time more fun for everyone.

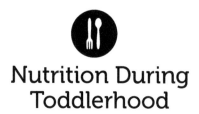

Nutrition During Toddlerhood

It is **obvious,** toddlers can be picky eaters.

One of the biggest concerns parents have about their toddlers is their sporadic eating patterns. From "He won't eat anything," to "All she does is snack," trying to get good nutrition into your toddler can be a challenge.

By the age of one, most kids should be eating what you eat, with a picky preference here and there. They may still be eating some pureed foods and taking milk out of a bottle, but they are learning how to eat a variety of foods independently and are starting to drink out of some type of cup.

It is important to get rid of the bottle before the age of two. Prolonged bottle use can increase the risk of sleep problems, weight gain and tooth decay. Most children transition from formula or breast milk to whole cow milk or a milk alternative at around 12 months of age. After 12 months of age, milk is more of a supplement than the main source of nutrition. There are many cow milk alternatives that are fortified, so if you are vegan, vegetarian, or your child isn't tolerating cow milk, try another alternative such as soy milk, almond milk, or coconut milk. Keep in mind that, as with cow milk, they all have a fairly high amount of sugar and therefore should be limited to less than 20 ounces per day.

You can start having them drink water when they are thirsty as well. Avoid or limit juice to four to six ounces per day to decrease sugar and the need for a sweet taste, and try not to give your children soft drinks! They aren't good for you and they're even worse for children of all ages.

Toddlers are usually too busy to sit for long periods during meals, so split the meals up or give them healthy snacks on the run. Avoid too many processed snacks, and switch up their snack choices. Fruits and vegetables are great snacks and more nutritious then processed crackers and fruit chews. Enjoy your snacks and meals together when possible. Show your love of nutritious food.

Give your toddler a child-safe utensil to practice with, but also let them use their fingers to eat. Remember they are still learning and are going to make a mess of the area around them. Limit foods with high salt and/or sugar content because those foods can be more addictive and will overpower the natural taste of less processed foods. Due to the varying amounts of food toddlers eat and their pickiness, you may have to look at their nutritional intake by the day or week rather than each meal.

Monkey see, monkey do: Your children learn by watching you, so be conscious about your eating habits. Avoid eating while watching TV or looking at your phone. Eat your vegetables first to prime your system and to show your children how good they are. Express gratitude for your food. Show respect for your food by controlling portion size and limiting the amount of food you throw away.

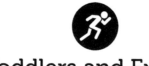

Toddlers and Exercise

You will **obviously** be on the move raising a toddler!

Once toddlers start walking, your body will have to be on the move just to keep up with them. You will definitely get your daily 10,000 steps in by raising an active toddler. Show them you enjoy moving with them.

Try to limit family TV time. This is a perfect time to become a more moving, rather than sitting family. Developmentally it is important that toddlers learn how to use their lower and upper bodies together by throwing a ball or by climbing.

This can be a trickier time to do your own movement activity because toddlers don't like being strapped in a stroller or carriage for too long. Don't give up! Show your children the pleasure it brings to move the way you want to, but lower your expectations about how far or long you can do it with them. Toddlers love watching and playing with their parents while they work out at home.

Toddlers and Spirituality

It is **obvious** that your toddler is a free spirit!

As their confidence builds, toddlers start exploring and pushing the boundaries of the physical and emotional world. Toddlers remind us how fun it is to feel free and explore new things. A free spirit doesn't mean there shouldn't be discipline and order in the home. Children thrive with structure and order, and need to know their boundaries.

Toddlers seem to have a never-ending supply of energy which means you need to keep your energy up too. Take turns with your partner so each of you can have some time alone to relax, exercise, or work on your personal goals. Learn to take deep and centering breaths, especially when you or your toddler are tired and your toddler pushes your buttons.

With toddlerhood, communication starts to become a two-way street. Talk to your children about gratitude, respect, and love. Show them the power of expressing gratitude when they are enjoying something. Read to them about the wonder of diversity. Teach them how to respect everyone no matter the color of their skin, their gender, or their ethnic background.

When speaking to your toddler, get down to their level and look them in the eyes. Hug them frequently, and say, "I love you" more than once a day. Giving children your undivided attention is one of the best gifts you can bestow upon them.

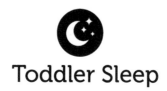

Toddler Sleep

Obviously we all deserve a good night's sleep!

If you are lucky, your toddler will be sleeping through the night. Unless your provider tells you otherwise, try to avoid feeding your child from the breast or bottle in the middle of the night to reduce the risk of cavities and the need for food as a soothing tool. Your toddler should start to be able to fall asleep without having a bottle or breast in their mouth.

There is no hurry to transition your toddler from a crib to a bed unless they are risking injury by jumping out of the crib or asking to sleep in a "big kid bed." Most toddlers move out of the crib by four years old, but they can be older if they like their crib. Talk to them about the transition to a bed before it happens. This includes discussing rules about their new freedom.

Most toddlers need a little "chill" time before falling asleep. Continue a bedtime routine that may involve reading, snuggling, singing, or listening to nice soft music with you. This is a great opportunity to have one-on-one time with your toddler. Most toddlers prefer to have a night-light on but make sure it is not too bright. Our brains need darkness to release melatonin to help trigger sleep. Try not to fall asleep with them every night because they may become dependent on that.

Toddler Well-Care Visits

Parents of toddlers **obviously** need some support!

During toddlerhood and early adolescence, your child's physical growth should remain steady. Any drastic changes in growth will be picked up at the well-care visit and addressed. The normal set of vital measurements including height, weight, blood pressure, and a vision screen (starting at age three) will be performed. This is a good time to discuss development and some of the frustrations related to raising a toddler. Topics from potty training to how to deal with tantrums can be discussed. Risks of lead poisoning will be addressed, and if needed, a lead blood level will be ordered.

In general, toddlers are more exposed to diseases as they start daycare, preschool, and kindergarten. Expect your child to get sick more often during this time. It is common for them to have up to 12 different illnesses within a year after starting daycare or preschool. Just as you would expect other parents to keep a sick child home, please don't allow your contagious child to be around other children.

Vaccines are not only protecting your child but the children they are in contact with! Vaccines are not perfect, but they do reduce the risk of contracting a potentially serious disease. Talk to your provider about what ages the various vaccines are recommended. Again, educate yourself on why they are recommended, what the risks of refusing them are, and what the possible side effects are.

Vaccines are usually recommended at the 12-month, 15-month, and 18-month well-child visits. If you follow the recommended schedule, there may not be any vaccines due after the 18-month visit until your child is four years old. This doesn't include the yearly flu vaccine recommended each fall. After the booster vaccines are given at four or five years old, there is a gap until age 11 for scheduled vaccines (This is according to the 2016 recommended schedule).

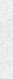

**WHERE TO FIND AN
UP-TO-DATE VACCINE SCHEDULE:**

www.healthychildren.org

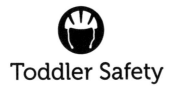

Toddler Safety

> **Obviously** you have your hands full, so try to have safety precautions already set in place.

Toddlerhood is one of the more difficult times to keep your child safe. Toddlers are always exploring and getting into things and do not yet understand caution. On a weekly basis I see at least one toddler escape the exam room and run down the hallway laughing, without a care in the world. As a parent, you have to walk that fine line between allowing natural consequences to happen and avoiding injury to your toddler.

Street Safety

Toddlers are small and quick and their actions are unpredictable. This makes playing around the street very dangerous. Toddlers are also hard for drivers to see, so keep an eye and hand on them around streets and parking lots. Teach them how to stop, look and listen for cars. Try to have them always cross at crosswalks with an adult. Use "slow down" or "children playing" signs on your street if needed. Make sure your toddler is always wearing a helmet when learning to ride a bike, scooter, or skateboard.

Car Safety

Keep your child rear-facing in their car seat until two years old if possible. They may fuss and say "I can't see" but the rear-facing position has proven to be safer. Toddlers may also want to use a seatbelt instead of a five-point harness because their older siblings and friends are using them. Remind your kids that super cool race car drivers all use a five-point seatbelt to stay safe. You can transition them into a booster seat using a seatbelt when they no longer fit in a five-point harness, are at least four years old and weigh around 40 pounds. When they transition to a seatbelt make sure it is not hitting their neck. Your kids should sit in the back seat, in the middle if possible, until they are around 13 years old.

In the House Safety

Make sure you have baby gates blocking the stairs if your child is not stable going up and down the stairs, but let them practice with your supervision. Make sure there are safety locks on all doors, cabinets and drawers that contain dangerous items. Do not make safety hazards a mystery. Toddlerhood is the time to start having conversations with your children about what is dangerous and what is safe. Children are less curious if they know the dangers.

Chemical Hazards (poisoning)

Some toxic liquids can look like a fun colored drink, so keep them out of sight and locked up. Other dangerous chemicals toddlers have been known to swallow include laundry and dishwasher detergent packets and button batteries, so keep those locked up as well. But again, show them what they look like and teach them not to touch or try to taste them.

Electrical Hazards

Teething toddlers like to chew on all sorts of things, including cords, so keep cords tucked away if possible. Cover all electrical outlets to prevent toddlers from sticking small metal objects (like your car keys) into them.

Burns

Hot water is the biggest cause for burns in infants and toddlers. Be careful with boiling water in the kitchen. Turn pot handles inward so your child can't reach up and grab them. Protect your toddler from other hot objects including fireplaces, open engine motors, and vaporizers.

Water (drowning)

A young child can drown in only a few inches of water. Watch them around any significant standing water including baths, pools, and even buckets of water. Most toddlers love to play with and in water. This is a great time to start teaching them water safety, which can include enrolling them in swim lessons. You and your infant can take swim lessons together, but most kids will not understand the concept of swimming until around age four. Dress your toddlers in bright-colored swimwear to make them more visible in the water.

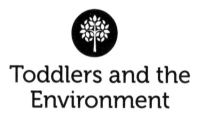

Toddlers and the Environment

It is **obvious** that most toddlers are curious creatures.

Toddlers have fewer opinions about what is gross or scary in the natural world. This is awesome! Have them explore nature by getting outside as much as possible. Show them different landscapes. Let them play with dirt and bugs but keep an eye on them because they still like to put things in their mouths! Encourage them to use their senses: to smell everything; feel changing temperatures outside; see a full moon after bedtime; listen to different bird calls; taste snowflakes they catch on their tongue; play in the rain; and get blown by the wind.

Toddlers are like little sponges, ready to soak up all sorts of knowledge, good or bad. Start talking to them about how to take care of Mother Earth. Teach them how to conserve water, but let them play with it (fill a basin for them to splash in, rather than letting them play with running water). Teach them how to turn off lights if they can reach the switch. Show them how to recycle and how to dispose of trash properly. Plant a garden with them and let them help take care of it. Let them eat straight from a vegetable garden. Teach them about all the other creatures we share the earth with. Explain to them why all creatures are an important part of the web of life.

MY OBVIOUS PARENTING PLAN
for Toddlerhood

Notes

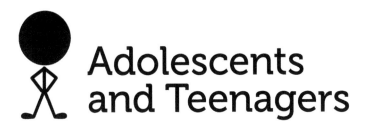

Adolescents and Teenagers

You **obviously** want to raise a respectful young man or woman.

This is a time when your kids give you a glimpse into their future selves, as they try out different roles and characters. One moment they are a loving, cuddly kid and the next moment they are an independent know-it-all. This can be frustrating for parents as we try to adapt our expectations to these changing behaviors. But we have to remember they are still kids. Step back and recall what troubles you gave your parents at this age!

Nutrition in Adolescents and Teenagers

> **Obviously** you want your growing children to make the right food choices.

We hope that some good eating habits have set in by this age. There is a natural progression to more independence in what they eat and the choices they have. You will have to trust they will make decent food choices when they are not around you. As a parent, be an anchor of good nutrition. Continue to try your best at eating healthy, remembering they are still watching you even though they will not admit it. Do not be a hypocrite; your kids will call you out on it! Keep your home stocked with more nutritional snack choices and avoid buying too much junk food even though your kids may beg for it.

Make it a priority to eat together at least once a day. Families that eat together stay closer together. Some teenagers have a tendency to stop eating breakfast and start eating late night snacks. Remind them that breakfast is important to kick start their metabolism and that late night snacks can affect sleep and increase calorie storage in the form of fat.

There is a significant amount of physical growth and foundation building during the adolescent and teenage years. Do you want your child's foundation to be built on sugar, salt, and fried fat? Do you want your already moody teenager to have "hangry" moments because they are consuming too much sugar? Of course you don't, so teach them the importance of eating more natural foods filled with fiber that helps regulate sugar absorption.

Be sure they are getting plenty of protein and complex carbohydrates to help fuel their growing muscles. Plants are a great source of protein and have 100 percent more fiber than meat. A diet high in fruits and vegetables has also been shown to help out with acne and other skin related issues that can be embarrassing for kids at this age.

Exercise for Adolescents and Teenagers

Obviously you want your children
to feel good about their bodies!

As your kids get older they will start keeping up with you, or even become faster and stronger then you are. It is awesome to see them develop physically. Try to keep up with them if you can and include them in your physical activities. Be open to attempting new activities that your kids are interested in. It seems that the times you are active with your kids are the times you bond better and remember more. Maybe it is the endorphins that help capture a strong memory and balanced outlook. Encourage your children to hang around active friends. If they are surrounded by movement they will move too.

Unfortunately, over-use injuries are becoming more common as kids only focus on one or two sports early in their lives. The increasingly competitive nature of organized sports can create extra stress on their bodies and minds while they are still developing. Let your children experience a variety of sports before committing to just one or two. Make sure they are focusing on the right techniques, stretches, and strengthening exercises to prevent chronic injuries.

As a general rule, if an activity continues to hurt, don't do it. It is fine to miss a few games in order to heal. Preventing chronic injuries now will allow them to keep getting better later. And most importantly, make sure they are having fun!

The teenage years are a wonderful age for our children to develop a body structure they would want to keep the rest of their lives. Allow your teenager to take advantage of the hormone changes in their bodies that can help build muscle mass and strength. You do not need a gym membership to stay fit. Using their own body weight for strength and conditioning is safe and easy. A few examples of exercises that can be done anywhere include pushups, lunges, pull-ups and core exercises. Muscles help increase metabolism making it more difficult to become overweight. Remind your children that movement that gets them breathing hard will help with focus, sleep, hormone balance, and bone strength.

Spirituality in Adolescents and Teenagers

It may not be **obvious**, but spirituality
can help bully-proof your child.

It can be hard for some kids to believe in any "higher power" even though it is within all of us. Continue to remind them they are never alone physically or spiritually. Remind them the only thing that matters is what they truly feel about themselves. The opinions and judgments of others should not affect their love for themselves.

Optimism

Start their day with a hot cup of optimism. While eating breakfast or in the car going to school, talk about how good the day is going to be, but be realistic about their current struggles. The true and only controller of our internal mood is ourselves, not external circumstances.

Service

The tweens and teens are a great age to find something they enjoy that helps others. This can be anything from volunteer service, being part of a club at school, or a paid job. If you ask them, "How did it make you feel to help someone?" most of the time the answer will be, "It felt good."

Commitment

Commitment is best taught by example. Show your child how being dedicated to a cause or activity drives success. Success in your career, hobbies, and especially as a parent. Commit to spending time with your family and supporting their health and wellness. Discuss commitment to education and how having greater knowledge leads to greater possibilities.

Teenage years are a time of conflict between trying to fit in and being their own person. Show your kids that you will always be there for them and try your best not to be judgmental. These years will go by more smoothly if everyone is less judgmental and more respectful of themselves and others. Both you and your kids need to keep an open mind. Let natural consequences happen if needed, and don't back down on finding out what they are doing and thinking. Get to know their friends by inviting them over for dinner (growing kids enjoy free food!).

Make your family time more adventurous. Your children will be more likely to spend time with you if you spice it up. Keep pushing gratitude. Let them hear you say, "I am so thankful for...." on a daily bases. Remind them this is a magical time, and they can feel more of that magic by calming their minds and listening to their bodies. Light that spark of interest with self-improvement books. Some of the wonderful authors I have found include Deepak Chopra, Wayne Dyer, Dan Millman, Richard Bach, Don Miguel Ruiz, James Redfield, and Eckhart Tolle. Look for these and many other wise authors/speakers that can help guide us in this human journey.

Be conscious of what music they are listening to. Listen to music with them and talk to them about how the music makes them feel. Music is a wonderful tool for self-expression and is a wonderful way to bond with our children.

Sleep for Adolescents and Teenagers

It is **obvious** that most kids want to
stay up later the older they get.

As we grow up we tend to stay up later, sometimes compromising the amount of sleep we get. It is recommended that adolescents and teenagers get at least eight hours of sleep. Studies have shown that the longest living people sleep more and take naps. So let your children sleep in on weekends and take naps to help balance the lack of sleep that occurs during the school week. Lacking quality sleep can increase blood pressure, decrease immune system function, and increase lack of focus and irritability. A higher proportion of growth hormone is released while sleeping, so remind your children that sleep is important for their growth.

Avoid nighttime distractions. Electronic devices like computers, tablets, and phones should be turned off through the night and preferably stored at a central family charging station outside the bedroom. Any backlit electronics may decrease the release of melatonin (sleep hormone) making it harder to fall asleep or stay asleep. Electronics also keep our minds going, especially if we are communicating with others. If your older children are having a hard time falling asleep, teach them how to focus only on their body and breathing, in a dark, quiet and cool bedroom.

Well-Care Visits for Adolescents and Teenagers

It is **obvious** our kids go through many physical and mental changes during adolescent and teenage years.

Yearly checkups during these ages are so important due to all the changes that occur. From developing independence to going through puberty, a lot is going on in your child's life. Checking in on their growth, development and stressors is an important preventative measure.

Late adolescence and teenage years are a good time to talk about risky behaviors and their potential consequences. If teens are sexually active, a screening test for sexually transmitted diseases (STD) is recommended on a yearly basis. Most STDs can be asymptomatic and teenagers are not the best about being open to their parents or others about their sexual activity. Checking their blood pressure, heart rate, and cholesterol levels may also be part of the visit, especially if there is a family history of heart disease.

All the physical and social changes can be very stressful for kids at this age so screening for depression and anxiety may also be recommended. These visits can be a good time for your teenager to talk privately with a health care provider about concerns they are not comfortable sharing with their parents.

Vaccines

The recommended vaccine schedule includes three different vaccines from 11 to 18 years old. These vaccines include Tdap, Meningitis, and HPV. There may be more vaccines recommended for foreign travel, so check with the CDC and your provider if you are planning to travel overseas. Your children should also get the seasonal influenza vaccine annually. It is never too late to catch up on vaccines if needed.

Tdap: Helps protect from tetanus and pertussis (whooping cough). Recent evidence shows the effectiveness of the pertussis portion of the vaccine decreases around 50 percent after three to five years. Check with your provider to determine when the booster is recommended. The current recommendation is every ten years.

Meningitis: Helps protect us from bacteria that can cause inflammation of the lining of the brain and spinal cord. If the inflammation is severe enough it can lead to permanent brain damage and death. Children will need to get a booster in three to five years if given this vaccine before 16 years old. Studies show your child is just as likely to get meningitis during the teenage years as they are during college. This is why it is now recommended to start this vaccine at 11 years old. Fortunately, bacterial meningitis is a rare disease.

HPV (human papilloma virus): This is really an anti-cancer vaccine. The virus it protects us from is the number one cause of cervical cancer and is a trigger for other cancers including esophageal, anal, and penile cancers. Recent evidence shows that HVP infections are decreasing in the vaccinated and unvaccinated populations, hopefully decreasing cancer rates as well.

Safety for Adolescents and Teenagers

It is **obvious** you do not want your more independent child to find themselves in a life or death situation!

Car accidents are the number one killer of teens and young adults! Cars are starting to become cool to kids at this age because they are getting closer to driving them or are already learning to drive.

Cars may be cool, but they can also be very dangerous and need to be respected. Follow all of the laws and rules that help protect us including seat belt use and the *graduated driver licensing program**.

Your vehicle also needs to be properly maintained to stay safe. This includes checking tire wear and pressure, headlights, and brakes.

Set a good driving example and show your kids how to respect the amount of concentration it takes to drive safely:

○ Do not text and drive

○ Do not drink and drive

○ Avoid road rage

○ Don't drive if you are tired or sleep deprived

***Graduated driver licensing (GDL) program:** A state-regulated program designed to help teenage drivers gain driving experience in a safer and more gradual manor to help reduce motor vehicle accidents. Most programs involve limiting the number of teenagers in the car, driving after dark, and increasing the amount of supervised driving time.

Homicide is one of the top four causes of death at this age. Teach your kids to be aware of their surroundings and listen to their gut. It is easy to be in the wrong place at the wrong time, especially if you are hanging around the wrong people. Help your teenager figure out who could be a "wrong person" by getting to know their friends. Being under the influence of drugs or alcohol can also help land them in a "not so safe" situation. As parents, we should continue to promote self-confidence and discuss peer pressure and its possible consequences.

Inside the Home

Due to the increased curiosity and strong drive for experimentation in the late adolescent and teenage years it is important to continue practicing home safety. As we allow more independence there will be more non-supervised time for them to get into things. Continue to keep all hazardous chemicals and medication locked up. Remind your teenager about the dangers of experimenting with fire. Teach them how to safely use cutting tools including knives and power tools.

Gun Safety

Whether you own a gun or not, educate yourself and your family about gun safety. Our children should not be handling a gun of any type without parent supervision. I recommend not having a firearm in the house if you have a depressed teenager at home. A determined teenager may be able to find a way to get into the gun safe and a firearm is a fast and very effective way to end a precious life. Remove this possibility sooner rather than later.

Outside the Home

As our kids get older they will sometimes act as though they are invincible. Keeping our kids active will help build strong bones, good body awareness and can help decrease serious injury. But remind them that if they fall while pushing their physical limits, it is going to hurt. Wearing PPE (personal protective equipment), especially helmets, is the cool thing to do. Let your children pick their own helmets out and personalize them with stickers, etc. Wear a helmet yourself! I see so many parents riding their bikes without helmets, leading their responsible helmet-wearing kids down a busy street. As with everything else, this is a wonderful opportunity for you to lead by example. Plus, most kids prefer parents without head injuries!

Water Safety

It is never too late to learn how to swim. Get them into swim lessons if you haven't already. Make sure they are using a life jacket when advised, including rafting, boating or open water swimming if they are not a strong swimmer.

Concussions

Concussion awareness has become a priority for the majority of contact sports. Growing evidence shows that repeated concussions can create permanent brain damage. Ask the coaches how they are teaching players to avoid concussions and what their policy is if your child gets a concussion. Make sure you, your kids, and their coaches do not rush getting them back into a contact sport or risky activity after a confirmed concussion. Would you rather your child be out for a few practices and games now, or have long-term neurologic and psychological consequences later from sustaining repeated concussions?

Follow the national Graduated Return to Play protocol as directed by your health care provider.

LEARN MORE ABOUT CONCUSSIONS:

www.concussiontreatment.com

Social Media

Social media will be an unavoidable part of your child's life. Being able to connect with people worldwide with the click of a button can be a wonderful thing, but it is also a growing cause of disconnect.

To truly connect with someone, you need to see them face to face because communication involves not only the spoken word but also body language. When protected behind a screen, people can be more cruel and insincere to each other.

Using an electronic device to communicate is also not real-time. Texting, Facebook messaging, etc. give kids the ability to take their time to think about their response instead of having a real-time conversation.

Already, we are seeing people lose the ability to read social cues because of their lack of face-to-face communication. Reinforce the need for face-to-face experiences with their friends and let them get together with their friends when possible.

Remind them that words spoken through social media can be deceiving. Talk to your children about avoiding negativity and gossip as much as possible. Make sure they understand that posting on social media can create a permanent record of their thoughts and activities.

Discuss cyber-bullying and the support you can give them if needed. A great thing about social media is that their phone, tablet or computer has an "OFF" switch and I recommend exercising your parental power and using that switch on a consistent basis to truly connect with your children.

TWO GOOD RESOURCES FOR SOCIAL MEDIA:

www.ncpc.org

www.esafety.gov.au

Environment in Adolescents and Teenagers

Teach your children the **obvious** truth that if we do not take care of our environment there will be serious consequences!

Your kids are now old enough to actively contribute to the good of the earth. Keep teaching them about the amazing natural world around them and give them the opportunity to learn by doing. Sign your family up to help clean parks and highways or help build trails. Around the house, let them start recycling and taking out the trash.

Have them investigate what power company you use to power your home and what resources it uses to produce energy. Show your teens how much it costs to power your home and determine what each of you can do to reduce that cost.

Discuss your household water usage and how you can reduce your consumption by taking shorter showers, installing efficient shower heads, and following your water company's recommended lawn-watering schedule.

Show your kids how to properly dispose of toxic chemicals and paints. Keeping your older children busy by exploring nature also helps limit screen time and boredom.

It is easier to appreciate nature if you get outside and truly experience it. Outdoor activities are a great way to spend one-on-one time with your children. Go on walks or bike rides with your children. Talk about fuel-efficient cars and public transportation with your teenagers. Let them look into what options besides the family car they can use to get around. Be a good role model and don't litter; that includes cigarette butts! Discuss global warming and its effects on our environment. When you plan a vacation, look into eco-tourism.

MY OBVIOUS PARENTING PLAN
for Adolescents & Teenagers

_____
_____
_____
_____

_____
_____
_____
_____

_____
_____
_____
_____

_____
_____
_____
_____

_____
_____
_____
_____

_____
_____
_____
_____

_____
_____
_____
_____

Notes

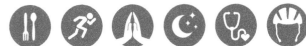

Conclusion

It is **obvious** that perfection is what you make of it.

Prevention is not perfect! There are so many factors in life that we can't control, but we can control the obvious ones. Get back to the basics. Slow down and take care of yourself and your family. Work together to keep your community healthy and safe. We all live on this planet together. To keep it running well, we need to respect everyone and everything on it, including ourselves.

Let us be grateful for life, and for our bodies and the ability to move and explore this world. Let us be grateful for our family and friends and the communities we live in. Let us be grateful for modern medicine and the tools it has blessed us with to stay healthy. Let us be grateful for nature's produce and having clean water to drink. Let us be grateful for sleep and its ability to recharge our bodies. Let us be grateful for learning from our mistakes and putting safety measures in place.

Let us be grateful for our faith in love and its ability to connect everyone and everything. Let us overcome our fear to give and receive love. Love is what will keep us working together. Let us keep fear from driving our decisions!

Let us support our health care system by putting less stress on it. We need to support wellness and try our best to stay healthy. We should use our health care system more for prevention and less for chronic illness.

Obvious parenting does not mean easy parenting. Try to keep convenience from controlling your health. When making decisions that will affect your family's health, think about the whole body, the whole earth, the magical web of life.

You could say, "Life is too short, live it up!" Or ask, "Why even try?" My response is this: Try because you have been given this wonderful vessel and earth to enjoy and respect. Do you want your children to grow up happy and healthy, living on a beautiful and clean planet? If so, let's join together and make wellness our obvious choice!

Thank You!

P.S. Thank your kids for allowing you to share in their journey!

Website Resources

Nutrition

Trans fats
- www.fda.gov/food/ucm292278.htm

Label reading
- www.fda.gov
- www.healthline.com

Basic Nutrition
- www.choosemyplate.gov
- https://my.clevelandclinic.org/articles/
  11208-fat-what-you-need-to-know

Dirty Dozen produce items with the highest pesticide levels
- www.ewg.org

What fish to eat and which fish are endangered
- www.nrdc.org
- www.safinacenter.org

Dairy
- www.pcrm.org

Exercise

Heart rate zones
- www.medicalnewstoday.com/articles/235710.php

Stretching
- www.mayoclinic.org
- www.bodybuilding.com

Sleep

Sleep safety

- www.nichd.nih.gov/sts/Pages/default.aspx
- www.healthychildren.org
- www.sleephealth.org

Well-Care Visits

Well-care schedule

- www.aap.org

Vaccine effectiveness

- www.vaccines.gov
- www.tycho.pitt.edu
- www.immunize.org/catg.d/p4037.pdf
- www.hhs.gov
- www.thescientificparent.org/vaccines-101-to-much-too-soon

Vaccine safety

- www.hrsa.gov
- www.who.int/vaccine_safety/initiative/tools/vaccinfosheets/en/
- www.cdc.gov/vaccine safety

Vaccine additives

- www.cdc.gov/vaccines/vac-gen/additives.htm
- www.publichealth.org

Oral health/water fluoridation

- https://ilikemyteeth.org/fluoridation
- www.aapd.org

Social Media

- www.ncpc.org
- www.esafety.gov.au

Safety

Car seats
- www.safecar.gov

Crib safety
- www.parents.com recall page

Concussion
- www.concussiontreatment.com

Environment

Quit smoking
- www.quitterscircle.com
- www.lung.org

Air pollution
- www.epa.gov
- www.niehs.nih.gov

Global warming
- https://climate.nasa.gov

Clean energy
- www.nrdc.org
- www.nrel.gov

Clean water
- www.nature.org
- www.greenfacts.org
- www.fao.org
- www.ewg.org
- www.cleanwateraction.org

Those other creatures
- www.worldwildlife.org
- www.nwf.org
- www.everythingconnects.org

About the Author

Ben Jessen is a father of two boys and a practicing physician assistant at a busy integrated pediatric office in Denver, Colorado. With more than fifteen years of experience in pediatrics, he has helped thousands of families to focus on a more holistic approach to healthcare. Ben feels strongly that prevention is the pillar to pediatric 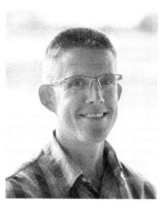 medicine and he continues to investigate and implement integrated methods of preventative care for his young patients as well as his own children.

Ben was born and raised in Colorado and enjoys spending time in the outdoors with his family. He truly practices what he preaches by keeping his own body and mind healthy so he can continue to make his wife and children crazy with his antics as long as possible!

www.ObviousParenting.com

email: *obviousparenting@gmail.com*